NURSING'S

SOCIAL POLICY STATEMENT

Second Edition

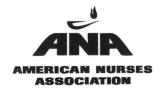

**AMERICAN NURSES
ASSOCIATION**

Silver Spring, MD

2003

Library of Congress Cataloging-in-Publication Data

American Nurses Association.
  Nursing's social policy statement / American Nurses Association.— 2nd ed.
      p. ; cm.
Includes bibliographical references and index.
  ISBN 1-55810-214-0
  1. Nursing. 2. Nursing—Philosophy. 3. Nursing—Practice. 4. Nursing—Social aspects.
  [DNLM: 1. Philosophy, Nursing. 2. Nurse's Role. 3. Nursing—standards. 4. Social Responsibility. WY 86 A512n 2003] I. Title.

  RT82.A59 2003
  610.73—dc22

                                   2003019622

Disclaimer: The American Nurses Association (ANA) is a national professional association. This ANA publication, *Nursing's Social Policy Statement, Second Edition*, reflects the thinking of the nursing profession on various issues relating to professional nursing practice and its relationship with society, its contribution to health care, and its obligation to those who receive nursing care. Thus, the contents of this book should be reviewed in conjunction with state board of nursing policies and practices. State law, rules, and regulations govern the practice of nursing, while *Nursing's Social Policy Statement, Second Edition* guides nurses in the application of their professional skills and responsibilities.

Published by Nursesbooks.org
The Publishing Program of ANA

American Nurses Association
8515 Georgia Avenue
Suite 400
Silver Spring, Maryland 20910-3492
1-800-274-4ANA (4262)
http://www.nursesbooks.org/

ANA is the only full-service professional organization representing the nation's 2.9 million Registered Nurses through its 54 constituent member associations. ANA advances the nursing profession by fostering high standards of nursing practice, promoting the economic and general welfare of nurses in the workplace, projecting a positive and realistic view of nursing, and by lobbying the Congress and regulatory agencies on healthcare issues affecting nurses and the public.

ISBN 13: 978-1-55810-214-9 ISBN-10: 1-55810-214-0 SAN: 851-3481
03NSPS 20M 03/07R
First printing September 2003. Second printing December 2004.
Third printing October 2005. Fourth printing March 2007.

CONTENTS

Preface

The ANA Congress on Nursing Practice and Economics is pleased to present the 2003 revision of the profession's social policy statement, the expression of the social contract between society and professional nursing in the United States of America. This document, created by registered nurses primarily to help them better understand this aspect of their profession, can inform others about the social context of professional nursing's contributions in healthcare.

Development of This Document

The review and revision of *Nursing's Social Policy Statement* (1995) involved thoughtful dialogue by many individuals occurring over several years. Members of the Congress on Nursing Practice and Economics helped create the direction and process for the work, some served diligently on the Task Force, but all brought insight, commitment, and thoughtful creativity to the consensus-building process. See Appendix A for the names of these individuals and a timeline showing the evolution of the three versions of this document. (The timeline also interleaves key dates in the closely related development of ANA's foundational standards of nursing practice and code of ethics for nurses.)

Moreover, hundreds of registered nurses in ANA organizational units, state nurses associations, and specialty nursing organizations throughout the country debated the contents of the document and provided written or verbal suggestions during the field review established to solicit widespread public comment. Truly, this statement reflects the synthesis of the best thinking of America's registered nurses.

In this revision, the Task Force recognized the importance of clearly identifying the recipients of professional nursing care, be they individuals, groups, families, communities, or populations. The terms *patient, client,* or *person* most often refer to individuals while *healthcare consumer* can represent an individual or group. To date, professional nursing has not yet selected *healthcare consumer* as the term best depicting the healthy or ill recipients of professional nursing care. Therefore, *patient* is used throughout the text to provide consistency and brevity. (For more details on this topic, see the discussion in Appendix A, Developing the 2003 Revision, page 22.)

Using This Document

Nursing's Social Policy Statement, Second Edition is a fundamental document that characterizes professional nursing and its social framework and obligations. This document, a keystone of the profession that supports the practice of all U.S. nurses, is closely related to two other ANA publications—*Code of Ethics for Nurses with Interpretive Statements* (2001) and *Nursing: Scope and Standards of Practice* (2003). Each document contributes in its own way to provide guidance to all nurses in their roles in education, supervision, administration, policy, research, and the provision of direct patient care.

Nursing's Social Policy Statement, Second Edition can be used by nurses to frame their understanding of professional nursing's relationship with society and its obligation to the recipients of professional nursing care. It can also inform others working in or involved with the healthcare industry about professional nursing's contribution. Healthcare consumers, as well as policy makers, legislators, employers, insurers, funding organizations, and others may gain insights for their decision-making.

Nursing's Social Policy Statement, Second Edition can be read and consulted on its own as both a standard reference text for all professional nursing practice, and as a standing companion volume to many educational and professional development activities. This revision offers several valuable appendixes. Instructors, students, scholars, and any others who are interested in how this fundamental document has evolved over the past 25 years will find Appendix A useful; it provides the context and some additional information on the development of this revision. Likewise, the full text of the 1980 and 1995 versions are included in Appendixes B and C, respectively.

This historical context is complemented by Appendix D, which includes definitions of nursing from two other organizations. These should help readers to better understand the new definition of professional nursing in the United States (see page 5) in a manner that better reflects practice here and abroad.

Nursing's Social Policy Statement, Second Edition now belongs to the profession. The Congress on Nursing Practice and Economics will monitor the use and critique of the 2003 statement, aware that the profession, health care, and society are constantly evolving. This ongoing work represents the profession's commitment to society and the people we serve.

Anne M. Hammes, MS, RN, CNAA
Chair, Congress on Nursing Practice and
Economics 2002–2004

Linda J. Gobis, JD, RN, FNP
Chair, Congress on Nursing Practice and
Economics 2000–2002

INTRODUCTION

"Nursing is <u>the</u> pivotal health care profession, highly valued for its specialized knowledge, skill and caring in improving the health status of the public and ensuring safe, effective, quality care. The profession mirrors the diverse population it serves and provides leadership to create positive changes in health policy and delivery systems. Individuals choose nursing as a career, and remain in the profession, because of the opportunities for personal and professional growth, supportive work environments and compensation commensurate with roles and responsibilities.[1]

The Social Context of Nursing

Nursing's Social Policy Statement, Second Edition expresses the social contract between society and the profession of nursing. Registered nurses and others can use this document as a framework for understanding professional nursing's relationship with society and its obligation to those who receive professional nursing care. It includes a definition of professional nursing, descriptions of professional nursing and its knowledge base, and brief descriptions of the scope of professional nursing practice and the methods by which the profession is regulated. These concepts underlie the practice of professional nursing, provide direction for clinicians, educators, administrators, and scientists within professional nursing, and inform other healthcare professionals, public policymakers, and funding bodies about professional nursing's contribution to health care.

This statement is derived from the 1980 landmark document, *Nursing: A Social Policy Statement,*[2] and *Nursing's Social Policy Statement,*[3] published in 1995. These documents provided the profession's earlier descriptions of its social responsibility and professional nursing's roles in the American healthcare system. The current document presents the practice of professional nursing as it has evolved, and provides direction for the future.

Professional nursing, like other professions, is an essential part of the society from which it grew and within which it continues to evolve. Professional nursing is dynamic, rather than static, reflecting the changing nature of societal needs. Professional nursing can be said to be owned by society, in the sense that "a profession acquires recognition, relevance, and even meaning in terms of its relationship to that society, its culture and institutions, and its other members."[4] This social contract between the broader society and its professions has been expressed as follows:

> Societies (and often vested interests within them)... determine, in accord with their different technological and economic levels of development and their socioeconomic, political and cultural conditions and values, what professional skills and knowledge they most need or desire... Logically, then, the professions open to individuals in any particular society are the property not of the individual but of the society. What individuals acquire through training is professional knowledge and skill, not a profession or even part ownership of one.[5]

The authority for the practice of professional nursing is based on a social contract that acknowledges professional rights and responsibilities as well as mechanisms for public accountability.

> Society grants the professions authority over functions vital to itself and permits them considerable autonomy in the conduct of their affairs. In return, the professions are expected to act responsibly, always mindful of the public trust. Self-regulation to assure quality in performance is at the heart of this relationship. It is the authentic hallmark of a mature profession.[6]

To maximize the contributions nurses make to society, it is necessary to protect the dignity and autonomy of nurses in the workplace. To that end, the American Nurses Association has adopted the *Bill of Rights for Registered Nurses.*[7]

Values and Assumptions of Nursing's Social Contract

The following values and assumptions undergird professional nursing's contract with society:

- Humans manifest an essential unity of mind, body, and spirit.
- Human experience is contextually and culturally defined.
- Health and illness are human experiences. The presence of illness does not preclude health nor does optimal health preclude illness.
- The relationship between nurse and patient involves participation of both in the process of care.
- The interaction between nurse and patient occurs within the context of the values and beliefs of the patient and the nurse.
- Public policy and the healthcare delivery system influence the health and well-being of society and professional nursing.

These values and assumptions apply whether the recipient of professional nursing care is an individual, family, group, community, or population.

DEFINITION OF NURSING

Definitions of nursing have evolved to acknowledge six essential features of professional nursing:

- provision of a caring relationship that facilitates health and healing,

- attention to the range of human experiences and responses to health and illness within the physical and social environments,

- integration of objective data with knowledge gained from an appreciation of the patient or group's subjective experience,

- application of scientific knowledge to the processes of diagnosis and treatment through the use of judgment and critical thinking,

- advancement of professional nursing knowledge through scholarly inquiry, and

- influence on social and public policy to promote social justice.

In her *Notes on Nursing: What It Is and What It Is Not*, published in 1859, Florence Nightingale defined nursing as having "charge of the personal health of somebody...and what nursing has to do...is to put the patient in the best condition for nature to act upon him."[8]

A century later, Virginia Henderson defined the purpose of nursing as "to assist the individual, sick or well, in the performance of those activities contributing to health or its recovery (or to a peaceful death) that he would perform unaided if he had the necessary strength, will or knowledge. And to do this in such a way as to help him gain independence as rapidly as possible."[9]

In the 1980 *Nursing: A Social Policy Statement*, nursing was defined as "the diagnosis and treatment of human responses to actual or potential health problems."[10]

A broader definition is consistent with professional nursing's commitment to meeting societal needs, and permits the profession and its practitioners to adapt to the ongoing changes in healthcare environments, practice expectations, and the profession itself. The evolution of nursing practice leads to the following definition of professional nursing:

> *Nursing is the protection, promotion, and optimization of health and abilities, prevention of illness and injury, alleviation of suffering through the diagnosis and treatment of human response, and advocacy in the care of individuals, families, communities, and populations.*[11]

Moreover, nursing addresses the organizational, social, economic, legal, and political factors within the healthcare system and society. These and other factors affect the cost, access to, and quality of health care and the vitality of the nursing profession. This is accomplished through a variety of means.

KNOWLEDGE BASE FOR NURSING PRACTICE

Nursing is a profession and a scientific discipline. The knowledge base for professional nursing practice includes nursing science, philosophy, and ethics, as well as physical, economic, biomedical, behavioral, and social sciences. To refine and expand the knowledge base and science of the discipline, nurses generate and use theories and research findings that are selected on the basis of their fit with professional nursing's values of health and health care, as well as their relevance to professional nursing practice.

Nurses are concerned with human experiences and responses across the lifespan. Nurses partner with individuals, families, communities, and populations to address issues such as:

- promotion of health and safety;
- care and self-care processes;
- physical, emotional, and spiritual comfort, discomfort, and pain;
- adaptation to physiologic and pathophysiologic processes;
- emotions related to experiences of birth, growth and development, health, illness, disease, and death;
- meanings ascribed to health and illness;
- decision-making and ability to make choices;
- relationships, role performance, and change processes within relationships;
- social policies and their effects on the health of individuals, families, and communities;
- healthcare systems and their relationships with access to and quality of health care; and
- the environment and the prevention of disease.

Nurses use their theoretical and evidence-based knowledge of these phenomena in collaborating with patients to assess, plan, implement, and evaluate care. Nursing interventions are intended to produce beneficial effects and contribute to quality outcomes. Nurses evaluate the effectiveness of their care in relation to identified outcomes and use evidence to improve care.

Scope of Nursing Practice

Professional nursing has one scope of practice, which encompasses the range of activities from those of the beginning registered nurse through the advanced level. While a single scope of professional nursing practice exists, the depth and breadth to which individual nurses engage in the total scope of professional nursing practice is dependent on their educational preparation, their experience, their role, and the nature of the patient population they serve.

Further, all nurses are responsible for practicing in accordance with recognized standards of professional nursing practice and professional performance. The level of application of standards varies with the education, experience, and skills of the individual nurse. Since 1965, ANA has consistently affirmed the baccalaureate degree in nursing as the preferred educational requirement for entry into professional nursing practice.[12] Each nurse remains accountable for the quality of care within his or her scope of nursing practice.

Professional nursing's scope of practice is dynamic and continually evolving. It has a flexible boundary that is responsive to the changing needs of society and the expanding knowledge base of its theoretical and scientific domains. This scope of practice thus overlaps those of other professions involved in health care. The boundaries of each profession are constantly changing, and members of various professions cooperate by sharing knowledge, techniques, and ideas about how to deliver quality health care. Collaboration among healthcare professionals involves recognition of the expertise of others within and outside the profession, and referral to those other providers when appropriate. Collaboration also involves some shared functions and a common focus on the same overall mission.

Nurses provide care for patients in a variety of settings. Nurses may initiate treatments or carry out interventions initiated by other authorized healthcare providers. Nurses are coordinators of care as well as caregivers.

Nursing practice includes, but is not limited to, initiating and maintaining comfort measures, promoting and supporting human functions and responses, establishing an environment conducive to well-being, providing health counseling and teaching, and collaborating on certain aspects of the health regimen. This practice is based on understanding the human condition across the life span and the relationship of the individual within the environment.

Nursing care is provided and directed by registered nurses and advanced practice registered nurses. All registered nurses are educated in the art and science of nursing with the goal of helping patients to attain, maintain, and restore health, or to experience a dignified death. Registered nurses and advanced practice registered nurses may also develop expertise in a particular specialty.

Specialization in Nursing

Specialization involves focusing on a part of the whole field of professional nursing. The American Nurses Association and specialty nursing organizations delineate the components of professional nursing practice that are essential for any particular specialty. Registered nurses may seek certification in a variety of specialized areas of nursing practice.

Advanced Practice Registered Nurses

Advanced practice registered nurses (that is, nurse practitioners, certified registered nurse anesthetists, certified nurse-midwives, and clinical nurse specialists) practice from both *expanded* and *specialized* knowledge and skills.

- *Expansion* refers to the acquisition of new practice knowledge and skills, including the knowledge and skills that authorize role autonomy within areas of practice that may overlap traditional boundaries of medical practice.

- *Specialization* is concentrating or delimiting one's focus to part of the whole field of professional nursing (such as ambulatory care, pediatric, maternal-child, psychiatric, palliative care, or oncology nursing).

Advanced practice is characterized by the integration and application of a broad range of theoretical and evidence-based knowledge that occurs as a part of graduate nursing education. Advanced practice registered nurses hold master's or doctoral degrees and are licensed, certified, and/or approved to practice in their roles.

Additional Advanced Roles

Continuation of the profession of nursing is also dependent on the education of nurses, appropriate organization of nursing services, continued expansion of nursing knowledge, and the development and adoption of policies consistent with values and assumptions that underlie the scope of professional nursing practice. Registered nurses may practice in such advanced roles as nurse educator, nurse administrator, nurse researcher, and nurse policy analyst. These advanced roles require specific additional knowledge and skills at the graduate level. Generally, those practicing in these roles hold master's or doctoral degrees.

Further details on the scope of professional nursing practice, specifics describing the *who, what, where, when, why,* and *how* of both specialized and advanced areas of nursing practice, are found in the current version of *Nursing: Scope and Standards of Practice.*[13]

THE REGULATION OF NURSING PRACTICE

Professional nursing, like other professions, is accountable for ensuring that its members act in the public interest in the course of providing the unique service society has entrusted to them. The processes by which the profession does this include self-regulation, professional regulation, and legal regulation.

Self-Regulation

Self-regulation involves personal accountability for the knowledge base for professional practice. Nurses develop and maintain current knowledge, skills, and abilities through formal and continuing education. Where appropriate, nurses hold certification in their area of practice to demonstrate this accountability.

Nurses also regulate themselves as individuals through peer review of their practice. Continuous performance improvement fosters the refinement of knowledge, skills, and clinical decision-making processes at all levels and in all areas of professional nursing practice. As expressed in the profession's code of ethics, peer review is one mechanism by which nurses are held accountable for practice

As noted in Provision 3.4 (Standards and Review Mechanisms) of *Code of Ethics for Nurses with Interpretive Statements*,[14] nurses should also be active participants in the development of policies and review mechanisms designed to promote patient safety, reduce the likelihood of errors, and address both environmental system factors and human factors that present increased risk to patients. In addition, when errors do occur, nurses are expected to follow established guidelines in reporting errors committed or observed.

Professional Regulation

Professional nursing defines its practice base, provides for research and development of that practice base, establishes a system for nursing education, establishes the structures through which nursing services will be delivered, and provides quality review mechanisms such as a code of ethics, standards of practice, structures for peer review, and a system of credentialing.

Professional regulation of nursing practice begins with the profession's definition of nursing and the scope of professional nursing practice. Professional standards are then derived from the scope of professional nursing practice.

Certification is a judgment of competence made by nurses who are themselves practicing within the area of specialization. Several credentialing boards are associated with the American Nurses Association and with specialty nursing organizations. These boards develop and implement certification examinations and procedures for nurses who wish to have their specialty practice knowledge recognized by the profession and the public. One component of the required evidence is successful completion of an examination that tests the knowledge base for the selected area of practice. Other requirements relate to the content of coursework and amount of supervised practice.

Legal Regulation

All nurses are legally accountable for actions taken in the course of professional nursing practice as well as for actions assigned by the nurse to others assisting in the provision of nursing care. Such accountability is accomplished through the legal regulatory mechanisms of licensure and criminal and civil laws.

The legal contract between society and the professions is defined by statute and by associated rules and regulations. State nurse practice acts and related legislative and regulatory initiatives serve as the explicit codification of the profession's obligation to act in the best interests of society. Nurse practice acts grant nurses the authority to practice and grant society the authority to sanction nurses who violate the norms of the profession or act in a manner that threatens the safety of the public.

Statutory definitions of nursing should be compatible with and build upon the profession's definition of its practice base, but be general enough to provide for the dynamic nature of an evolving scope of nursing practice. Society is best served when consistent definitions of the scope of nursing practice are used by states. This allows residents of all states to access the full range of nursing services.

CONCLUSION

Nursing's Social Policy Statement, Second Edition describes professional nursing in the United States of America. It includes an identification of the values and the social responsibility of the profession, a definition of professional nursing, a brief discussion of the scope of practice, and a description of professional nursing's knowledge base and the methods by which professional nursing is regulated. *Nursing's Social Policy Statement, Second Edition* provides both an accounting of nursing's professional stewardship and an expression of professional nursing's continuing commitment to the society it serves.

References

1. Nursing's Agenda for the Future Steering Committee. *Nursing's Agenda for the Future* (Washington, D.C.: American Nurses Publishing, 2001). Also available on the ANA web site: http://www.nursingworld.org/naf/

2. American Nurses Association. *Nursing: A Social Policy Statement* (Kansas City, MO. American Nurses Association, 1980).

3. American Nurses Association. *Nursing's Social Policy Statement* (Washington, D.C.: American Nurses Publishing, 1995).

4. Page, B.B. "Who owns the profession?," *Hastings Center Report* 5(5): 7–8 (1975).

5. Ibid., 7.

6. Donabedian, A. Foreword in M. Phaneuf, *The Nursing Audit: Self-Regulation in Nursing Practice*, 2nd ed. (New York: Appleton-Century-Crofts, 1972), 8.

7. American Nurses Association. *Bill of Rights for Registered Nurses* (Washington, D.C.: American Nurses Publishing, 2001), 1.

8. Nightingale, F. *Notes on Nursing: What It Is and What It Is Not.* (1859; reprint, New York: J. B. Lippincott Company, 1946), preface, 75.

9. Henderson, V. *Basic Principles of Nursing Care* (London: International Council of Nurses, 1961), 42.

10. American Nurses Association, *Nursing: A Social Policy Statement.* (Kansas City, MO. American Nurses Association, 1980).

11. Adapted from: American Nurses Association. *Code of Ethics for Nurses with Interpretive Statements* (Washington, D.C.: American Nurses Publishing, 2001), 5. (Also on the ANA web site: http://nursingworld.org/ethics/ecode.htm)

12. American Nurses Association House of Delegates. *Titling for Licensure* (Kansas City, MO: American Nurses Association, 1985).

13. American Nurses Association. *Nursing: Scope and Standards of Practice* (Washington, D.C.: American Nurses Publishing, 2003).

14. American Nurses Association, *Code of Ethics for Nurses with Interpretive Statements*, 13–14.

15. Ibid., 24.

Appendix A
The Development of Nursing's Social Policy Statements, 1980–2003

Contributors, 1980–2003

Nursing's Social Policy Statement Revision Task Force, 2001–2003
Naomi E. Ervin, RN, PhD, APRN, BC, FAAN; *Chair (2002–2003)*
Anne M. McNamara, PhD, RN; *Chair (2001–2002)*
Linda A. Beechinor, MS, RN, FNP
Joan M. Caley, RN, MS, CNAA, CS
Mary B. Killeen, PhD, RN, C, CNAA
Linda L. Olson, PhD, RN, CNAA
Susan Foley Pierce, PhD, RN
Steven R. Pitkin, RN, MN
Betty Smith-Campbell, PhD, RN, ARNP
Susan Tullai-McGuinness, PhD, MPA, RN
Marva Wade, RN

Social Policy Statement Task Force, 1992–1995
Linda R. Cronenwett, PhD, RN, FAAN; *Facilitator (1994–1995)*
Barbara E. Pokorny, MSN, RN, CS; *Facilitator (1992–1993)*
Kathryn Barnard, PhD, RN, FAAN
Susan E. Doughty, MSN, RN, CS
Beverly Hall, PhD, RN, FAAN
Gail A. Harkness, DrPH, RN, FAAN
Mary S. Koithan, PhD, RN
Frank R. Lamendola, MSN, RN, CS
Mary K. Walker, PhD, RN, FAAN

***Nursing: A Social Policy Statement*, Authors, 1980**
Norma Lang, PhD, RN, FAAN; *Chair*
Nina T. Argondizzo, MA, RN
Kathryn Barnard, PhD, RN, FAAN
Hildegard E. Peplau, EdD, RN, FAAN
Maria C. Phaneuf, MA, RN, FAAN
Jean E. Steel, PhD, RN, FAAN
Glenn Webster, PhD

Congress on Nursing Practice and Economics 2002–2004
Anne M. Hammes, MS, RN, CNAA; *Chair*
Marva Wade, RN, *Vice Chair*
Kathryn Ballou, PhD, RN
Joan M. Caley, MS, RN, CS, CNAA
Naomi E. Ervin, RN, PhD, APRN, BC, FAAN
Tracy A. Hollar-Ruegg, MS, RN, CNP
Saul Josman, MN, RN, APRN-BC
David Marshall, JD, RN, CNAA
Mary A. Maryland, PhD, APRN,BC , APN
Maureen Ann Nalle, PhD, RN
Susan Foley Pierce, PhD, RN
Steven R. Pitkin, RN, MN
Lorna Samuels, BSN, RN, BC
Cathalene Teahan, MSN, RN, CNS
Susan Tullai-McGuinness, PhD, MPA, RN

Congress on Nursing Practice and Economics 2000–2002
Linda J. Gobis, JD, RN, FNP; *Chair*
Anne M. McNamara, PhD, RN, *Vice Chair*
Linda A. Beechinor, MS, RN, FNP
Sharon Bidwell-Cerone, PhD, RN, CS-PNP
Joan M. Caley, RN, MS, CNAA, CS
Mary Chaffee, MS, RN, CNA, CCRN
Naomi E. Ervin, PhD, RN, CS, FAAN
Anne M. Hammes, MS, RN, CNAA
Saul Josman, MN, RN, APRN-BC
Mary B. Killeen, PhD, RN, C, CNAA
Patricia (Patti) J. Kummeth, MSN, RN, C
David Marshall, JD RN, BSN
Linda L. Olson, PhD, RN, CNAA
Steven R. Pitkin, RN, MN
Lorna Samuels, BSN, RN, C
Marva Wade, RN

ANA Staff
Mary Jean Schumann, MSN, RN, MBA CPNP
Carol J. Bickford, PhD, RN, BC
Rita Munley Gallagher, PhD, RN,C
Christine Byrams, BBA
Vernice A. Woodland, MA

Timeline of the Development of Foundational Nursing Documents

The American Nurses Association has long been instrumental in the development of three foundational documents for professional nursing—a code of ethics, the scope and standards of practice, and a social policy statement. Each document contributes to the understanding of the context of nursing practice at the time of publication and reflects the history of the evolution of the nursing profession in the United States. Advancing communication technologies have expanded the revision process to permit ever increasing numbers of registered nurses to contribute to the open dialogue and review activities. This ensures the final published versions not only codify the consensus of the profession at the time of publication, but also reflect the experiences of those working in the profession at all levels and in all settings.

1859   Florence Nightingale publishes *Notes on Nursing: What It Is and What It Is Not.*

1896   The Nurses' Associated Alumnae of the United States and Canada is founded. Later to become the American Nurses Association (ANA), its first purpose was to establish and maintain a code of ethics.

1940   A "Tentative Code" is published in the *American Journal of Nursing,* although never formally adopted.

1950   *Code for Professional Nurses,* in the form of 17 provisions that are a substantive revision of the "Tentative Code" of 1940, is unanimously accepted by the ANA House of Delegates.

1952   *Nursing Research* publishes its premiere issue.

1956   *Code for Professional Nurses* is amended.

1960   *Code for Professional Nurses* is revised.

1968   *Code for Professional Nurses* is substantively revised, condensing the 17 provisions of the 1960 Code into 10 provisions.

1973   ANA publishes its first *Standards of Nursing Practice.*

1976   *Code for Nurses with Interpretive Statements,* a modification of the provisions and interpretive statements, is published as 11 provisions.

1980   ANA publishes *Nursing: A Social Policy Statement.*

1985   The National Institutes of Health organizes the National Center for Nursing Research.

ANA publishes *Titling for Licensure.*

Code for Nurses with Interpretive Statements retains the provisions of the 1976 version and includes revised interpretive statements.

The ANA House of Delegates forms a task force to formally document the scope of practice for nursing.

Foundational Nursing Documents

1987   ANA publishes *The Scope of Nursing Practice.*

1990   The ANA House of Delegates forms a task force to revise the 1973 *Standards of Nursing Practice.*

1991   ANA publishes *Standards of Clinical Nursing Practice.*

1995   ANA publishes *Nursing's Social Policy Statement.*

1995   The Congress of Nursing Practice directs the Committee on Nursing Practice Standards and Guidelines to establish a process for periodic review and revision of nursing standards.

1996   ANA publishes *Scope and Standards of Advanced Practice Registered Nursing.*

1998   ANA publishes *Standards of Clinical Nursing Practice, 2nd Edition* (also known as the *Clinical Standards*).

2001   *Code of Ethics for Nurses with Interpretive Statements* is accepted by the ANA House of Delegates.

        ANA publishes *Bill of Rights for Registered Nurses.*

2002   ANA publishes *Nursing's Agenda for the Future: A Call to the Nation.*

2003   ANA publishes *Nursing's Social Policy Statement, 2nd Edition.*
        ANA publishes *Nursing: Scope and Standards of Practice.*

Developing the 2003 Revision: Notes on Terminology

In this revision, the 2001–2003 Work Group responded to the widespread suggestion that the document be both clear and brief. Two areas of compromise contributed to brevity but not always to precision.

First, the *collective* recipients of nursing care are individuals, groups, families, communities, and populations. This point is made frequently throughout this document, but not in every possible paragraph. We ask readers to keep in mind that the breadth of nursing practice always includes these various recipients of care.

Second, the *individual* recipient of nursing care can be referred to as *patient, client,* or *person.* Instead of using all terms or varying terms throughout the document, we chose to refer to individual recipients of care as *patients.*

We acknowledge that *client* is preferred by some nurses because it connotes a more egalitarian relationship than *patient. Client,* however, also implies that a choice can be made by the recipient of care about which professional, among many, will provide their desired services. At this point in our history, the bulk of nursing practice does not offer the recipient of care that type of choice. *Patient,* therefore, is used throughout the text to provide consistency and brevity, with the awareness that *client* or *individual* might, in some instances, be a better choice.

APPENDIX B
TEXT OF THE 1980 ORIGINAL:
NURSING: A SOCIAL POLICY STATEMENT

Reproduced in this appendix are the pages of *Nursing: A Social Policy Statement*, the 1980 initiating publication of ANA's social policy statements. Similarly, the 1995 revision, *Nursing's Social Policy Statement*, is reproduced in Appendix C, which starts on page 59.

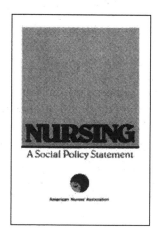

Contents

Preface

During 1979 the Committee of Chairpersons of the American Nurses' Association adopted as a goal the development of a coherent policy on nursing resources and coordinated strategy for implementation of the policy, including appropriate credentialing and establishment of qualifications for entry into nursing practice. A series of program activities were proposed to achieve that goal. The chairpersons determined that the Congress for Nursing Practice should assume responsibility for defining the nature and scope of nursing practice, including a description of the characteristics of specialization in nursing. The intent of the chairpersons was that the completed document serve as the basis for ANA policy.

The Congress for Nursing Practice is the structural unit of the American Nurses' Association charged by the Bylaws with responsibility for activities dealing with the scope of nursing practice, legal aspects of nursing practice, public recognition of the significance of nursing practice to health care, and the implications for nursing practice of trends in health care.

To accomplish this work, the Congress for Nursing Practice appointed a seven-member task force. The congress acknowledges the significant contributions to the advancement of nursing practice made by the task force, and expresses its particular appreciation of the contributions to that group by Hildegard Peplau and Maria Phaneuf. Their distinguished careers have helped to shape the nursing profession, and their continuing commitment to the profession is demonstrated by their indispensable participation in the work of the task force.

The Congress for Nursing Practice is indebted to the ANA Divisions on Practice and practice councils, and to the many other nurses, both individuals and groups, who reviewed and commented on a draft of this statement circulated in June 1980. To those nurses who attended the forum on the draft held at the ANA biennial convention in Houston, Texas, in June 1980, and to those who responded verbally or in writing to the draft, the congress expresses its gratitude for the interest and insights they shared.

The congress also acknowledges its appreciation of the work of ANA staff in preparation of the statement, especially that of Katherine Goldring, editor of publications, and Ruth Lewis, director of the Nursing Practice Department.

Norma Lang, Ph.D., R.N., F.A.A.N.
Chairperson
American Nurses' Association
Congress for Nursing Practice

Introduction

During the last century, the question, "What is nursing?" has been raised by nurses as well as by other health professionals, legislators, and the public. During these years, nursing has steadily responded by moving forward in its conception of its work in consonance with evolving professional and social demands. Trends well under way in nursing must now be reflected in a contemporary delineation of the nature and scope of nursing practice and a description of the characteristics of specialization in nursing.

As the professional society for nursing in the United States, the American Nurses' Association is responsible for defining and establishing the scope of nursing practice. Publication of this statement enhances ongoing professional dialogue and contributes to the work of nursing's professional society in carrying out its responsibility.

The statement includes emphasis on specialization because the development of specialization in nursing practice has been a major advance in nursing during the last three decades. The profession is therefore obliged to provide means of identifying within nursing and for the public those nurses who meet stipulated criteria as specialists, so as to assure the public that those nurses who present themselves as specialists are so qualified.

The nursing profession has reached a maturity that not only justifies but also requires a statement affirming nursing's social responsibility, made in recognition of society's right to know how that responsibility is exercised in nursing practice. The nature and scope of nursing practice and characteristics of specialization in nursing have therefore been delineated here in a social policy statement.

This statement is intended as a fundamental and undergirding delineation, providing a foundation that promotes unity in nursing in a basic and common approach to practice. The statement presents facts and values in nursing as they govern relationships to the larger professional and social context. It provides enabling definitions and descriptions, seeking to clarify the direction in which nursing has evolved and to provide a means for distinguishing between desirable and undesirable directions for future development. It is hoped that this formulation of nursing's social responsibility will further the growth of the profession and the development of nursing theory.

This delineation of the nature and scope of nursing practice is tailored to the diversity, openness, and transition characteristic of the present, actual range of nursing practice. Attempts to conceptually delimit nursing more clearly than it is actually delimited would have been potentially harmful. Such attempts would not only have been unjust to many nurses, but could be used prematurely or arbitrarily to limit the scope of nursing practice; care has been taken to avoid both of these pitfalls.

The statement is intended for use by nurses in achieving a fresh perspective on their practice, in helping the profession to move forward at a speed consistent with soundness and based on the achievements already attained, and in giving society a current view of the nature of nursing practice.

Useful as definitions and descriptions may be, they cannot accomplish what only political processes can achieve. Neither definitions nor descriptions can determine the actual scope of practice over the years ahead. Nor can they determine the relationships within nursing, between nursing and other health professions, between nursing and the various publics it serves, or between nursing and governmental bodies that formulate and direct implementation of public policy pertinent to health care systems, including the education of health professionals. It is individuals and groups working together through political processes who make these determinations. Because this social policy statement on the nature and scope of nursing practice, including its description of the characteristics of specialization in nursing, attests to nursing's social responsibilities, use of it by the individuals and groups who make the determinations that influence current developments and the shape of the future is essential.

The 1980s have been identified as a decade of decision in nursing. The social policy statement has been so cast as to facilitate decisions through which nursing can consolidate achievements of the past and move with wisdom and courage into its future of service to society.

I. The Social Context of Nursing

Nursing, like other professions, is an essential part of the society out of which it grew and with which it has been evolving. Nursing can be said to be owned by society, in the sense that nursing's professional interest must be and must be perceived as serving the interests of the larger whole of which it is a part. The mutually beneficial relationship between society and its profession has been expressed as follows:

> A profession acquires recognition, relevance, and even meaning in terms of its relationship to that society, its culture and institutions, and its other members. Professions acquire recognition and relevance primarily in terms of needs, conditions, and traditions of particular societies and their members. It is societies (and often vested interests within them) that determine, in accord with their different technological and economic levels of development and their socioeconomic, political and cultural conditions, and values, what professional skills and knowledge they most need and desire. By various financial means, institutions will then emerge to train interested individuals to supply those needs.

> Logically, then, the professions open to individuals in any particular society are the property not of the individual but of society. What individuals acquire through training is professional knowledge and skill, not a profession or even part ownership of one.[1]

Some Current Social Concerns and Directions in Health Care

Health care is currently a major focus of attention in the United States. Public and political determinations are being made in five major areas, in each of which nursing has leadership responsibilities:

1. Organization, delivery, and financing of health care. Attention to this area has been sharpened by the costs of care, which threaten to rise beyond the finite national economic capabilities, and by a public morality that requires a general availability, accessibility, and acceptability of health care.

2. Continuing development of health resources, including facilities and manpower for personal care and community health services, in a manner consistent with available knowledge and technology, and an increasing focus on individuals, families, and other groups as basic self-help resources.

3. Provision for the public health through use of preventive and environmental measures, and increased assumption of responsibility by individuals, families, and other groups as basic self-help resources.

4. Development of new knowledge and technology through research.

5. Health care planning as a matter of national policy and related regulations, made specific by the National Health Planning and Resources Development Act of 1974 (Public Law 93-641).

In these and other areas, public determinations find expression through political processes carried out by governmental and voluntary bodies. The political process includes the identification of public needs and demands and of the resources available to meet them, combined with appropriation and allocation of funds to support the resources. The political process also can be and is used to shape public perceptions of needs, and thus to create public demands. At best, such use of the political process is made out of impartial concerns for the public good. At worst, it occurs for the advancement of vested interests, with the public good being of lesser or no concern. For nursing, the public good must be the overriding concern.

Through political channels in our democracy, public determinations in the five areas previously mentioned are being made in a time of transition from a disease-oriented to a health-oriented system of health care. The transition is occurring in part because of the rising costs of hospital and related medical care. When the costs of the care of the sick rise so strikingly, questions are raised about the possibility of reducing costs by preventing or controlling disease or illness by focusing on attaining, maintaining, and regaining health.

Transition from a disease-oriented to a health-oriented system of care is an evolutionary process; such processes occur over time, at a slow pace, and they are often characterized by some denial that change is occurring or that it is even possible. Health care planning as a matter of national policy is evidence that change to a health-oriented system has at least been initiated. This new focus is symbolized by the use of the words *health care* in place of *medical care* and by the increasing use of the term *health center* for hospital. The newly perceived importance of ambulatory care, primary care, and family care centers, home health services, and other patterns of care, the increasing utilization of such types of care, and the provision of public and private payment for it clearly show the impact of the evolving health orientation.

While the health orientation can help to prevent, modify, or limit disease or illness, it cannot eliminate them. This change in approach in no way detracts from professional or institutional responsibility for care of the sick. In the movement to a health-oriented system of care, care of the sick remains a basic responsibility.

What is equally important is the growing realization that individuals, families, and groups have considerable responsibility for their personal health and for development of their potentials for achieving it. A public increasingly knowledgeable about health and health care systems is becoming more and more involved in related public and political decisions.

The decisions to come will be influenced by experience during the past two decades. The decade of the 1960s was characterized by the national spending of health care dollars without interfering in any way with the existing structure of the health care system. The decade of the 1970s was an era of new regulations designed to control the financial obligations resulting from the spending in the sixties. Regulation in its various forms was expensive, poorly designed, and largely ineffective.[2]

It is logical to anticipate that the 1980s will be a decade of increasing regulations with regard to the quantity, costs, and quality of health care. Because these elements are inextricably interwoven, increased attention will be concentrated on social and political options in health care. The development of social and political priorities for action will depend on choice among options, based on society's values and its needs.

Selected Specific Areas of Concern to Nursing

Nursing helps to serve society's interests in the area of health. The nursing profession has made and continues to make a substantial contribution toward evolution of a health-oriented system of care. Nursing practice has been health-oriented for more than half a century, partly because of its focus on individuals as persons and on the family as the necessary unit of service. In nursing so practiced, the current health movement was foreshadowed.

Health is a dynamic state of being in which the developmental and behavioral potential of an individual is realized to the fullest extent possible. Each human being possesses various strengths and limitations resulting from the interaction of environmental and hereditary factors. The relative dominance of the strengths and limitations determines an individual's place on the health continuum; it determines the person's biological and behavioral integrity, his wholeness.[3]

During periods of illness, trauma, or disability, an individual or family may require varying degrees of personal assistance in coping with a manifest problem, with the treatment plan designed to alleviate the problem, or with the sequelae. An individual or family may require varying degrees of assistance to obtain information in matters of health, to receive anticipatory guidance and therapeutic counseling to resolve problems, or to manage usual health practices, both during periods of wellness and when faced with a progressive or long-term health problem.

Viewed in this light, health becomes the center of nursing attention, not as an end in itself, but as a means to life that is meaningful and manageable.[4] Professional practice entails recognition that:

> Man has an inherent capacity for change in constructive and destructive directions. Access to opportunities for growth and possible change is every person's right, regardless of social or economic status, personal attributes, or the nature of the health problems. . . . Individual differences influence not only a person's potential for change, but also the meanings and values associated with it. Helping services that are founded on respect for human dignity recognize possibilities for individual freedom of choice and enhance opportunities for conscious self direction.[5]

A Nursing View of Working Relationships in Health Care

The nursing profession is particularly concerned with the working relationships essential to the carrying out of its health-oriented mission. The complexity and size of the health care system and its transitional state, increasing public involvement in health policy and a national focus on health, and the professionalization of nursing—all of these factors combine to intensify the importance of the direct human interactions inherent in nursing's response to human needs and society's expectations.

Nursing involvement in these interactions needs to be carried on with explicit assessment of the nature of working relationships. Conceptually there are three basic types of working relationships.[6] The first and most primitive is the one in which one person commands another. The second type can be identified as detente. The third level is collaboration.

In the first type, the person with power gives the command, which another obeys. In so commanding, the assumption is usually made that little knowledge, few skills, and little or no judgment or initiative are entailed in responding to the command. In health care, that assumption is generally false; the human beings involved have the capacity to exercise judgment, as warranted by the relevant knowledge and skills. This first level is essentially the master-slave relationship.

Detente implies power on both sides that is recognized by both, a recognition and acceptance of separate spheres of activity and responsibility, reciprocal acceptance of the legitimate interests of both parties, and some mutuality of interests and commonality of goals that are recognized by both parties. Detente may be likened to armed neutrality. It is a little-acknowledged prerequisite to genuine collaboration.

Collaboration means true partnership, in which the power on both sides is valued by both, with recognition and acceptance of separate and combined spheres of activity and responsibility, mutual safeguarding of the legitimate interests of each party, and a commonality of goals that is recognized by both parties. This is a relationship based upon recognition that each is richer and more truly real because of the strength and uniqueness of the other.

In practice, working relationships are rarely pure in type, even within individuals. Working relationships generally combine characteristics of the three types and vary with specific circumstances. In groups and in society as a whole there has been movement away from the command-obey type of relationship, through the detente type of interaction, toward collaboration, due to changes of a social and political nature affecting each of the health professions and the health care system. This change is part of the process of democratization that has been occurring for hundreds of years and has accelerated in the twentieth century.

Nursing must recognize and assess the nature of working relationships with patients and families, and with other health professionals and health workers, as well as relationships within nursing and between nursing and representatives of the public at large.

Authority for Nursing Practice

The authority for nursing, as for other professions, is based on a social contract, which in turn derives from a complex social base.

> There is a social contract between society and the professions. Under its terms, society grants the professions authority over functions vital to itself and permits them considerable autonomy in the conduct of their own affairs. In return, the professions are expected to act responsibly, always mindful of the public trust. Self-regulation to assure quality in performance is at the heart of this relationship. It is the authentic hallmark of a mature profession.[7]

As is necessary to a profession, nursing has a professional society—the American Nurses' Association — through which its responsibility to a society as a whole is exercised. Nursing's professional society performs an essential function in articulating and strengthening, as well as maintaining, the social contract that exists between nursing and society, upon which the authority to practice nursing is based.

That social contract has been made specific through the professional society's work derived from the collective expertise of its members, such as (1) establishing a code of ethics[8]; (2) establishing standards of practice[9]; (3) fostering development of nursing theory, derived from nursing research into those conditions that are the focus of practice, so as to explain observations and guide nursing actions; (4) establishing educational requirements for entry into professional practice[10]; (5) developing certification processes for the profession; and (6) other developmental work directed toward making more specific nursing's accountability to society.

One of the consequences of these and other of nursing's self-regulatory activities has been enactment of nursing practice acts and related licensure legislation and regulations that make specific the legal authority to practice. This legal authority to practice stems from the social contract between society and the profession; the social contract does not derive from legislation.

II. The Nature and Scope of Nursing Practice

A Definition of Nursing

In Nightingale's *Notes on Nursing: What It Is and What It Is Not*, published in 1859, nursing is defined as to have "charge of the personal health of somebody . . . and what nursing has to do . . . is to put the patient in the best condition for nature to act upon him."[11] A century later, Henderson defined nursing as "to assist the individual, sick or well, in the performance of those activities contributing to health or its recovery (or to a peaceful death) that he would perform unaided if he had the necessary strength, will or knowledge. And to do this in such a way as to help him gain independence as rapidly as possible."[12]

These definitions illustrate the consistent orientation of nurses to the provision of care that promotes well being in the people served. The nursing profession remains committed to the care and nurturing of sick and well people, individually and in groups.

The definition of nursing presented here maintains this historical orientation and at the same time reflects the influence of nursing theory that is a part of nursing's evolution:

Nursing is the diagnosis and treatment of human responses to actual or potential health problems.

This definition is based on language proposed in 1970 by the New York State Nurses Association.[13] This language was adopted as part of the Nurse Practice Act of New York State in 1972 and later incorporated in the nursing practice acts of several other states.[14, 15]

This definition points to four defining characteristics of nursing: phenomena, theory application, nursing action, and evaluation of effects of action in relation to phenomena.

Phenomena: The phenomena of concern to nurses are human responses to actual or potential health problems. Any observable manifestation, need, condition, concern, event, dilemma, difficulty, occurrence, or fact that can be described or scientifically explained and is within the target area of nursing practice is of interest to nurses. The human responses of people toward which the actions of nurses are directed are of two kinds: (1) reactions of individuals and groups to actual health problems (health-restoring responses), such as the impact of illness effects upon the self and family, and related self-care needs; and (2) concerns of individuals and groups about potential health problems (health-supporting responses), such as monitoring and teaching in populations or communities at risk in which educative needs for information, skill development, health-oriented attitudes, and related behavioral changes arise.

Nursing addresses itself to a wide range of health-related responses observed in sick and well persons. Those responses can be reactions to an actual problem, such as a disease, or they can anticipate a potential health problem. The difference between the response to a health problem and the problem itself is worth noting, as it is here where an intermeshing and complementarity of the distinct foci of the practices of nursing and medicine occur. Human responses to health problems, the phenomena to which the actions of nurses are directed, are often multiple, episodic, or continuous, fluid, and varying, and are less discrete or circumscribed than medical diagnostic categories tend to be.

The following provides an illustrative list rather than a comprehensive taxonomy of the human responses that are the focus for nursing intervention:

1. Self-care limitations

2. Impaired functioning in areas such as rest, sleep, ventilation, circulation, activity, nutrition, elimination, skin, sexuality, and the like

3. Pain and discomfort

4. Emotional problems related to illness and treatment, life-threatening events, or daily life experiences, such as anxiety, loss, loneliness, and grief

5. Distortion of symbolic functions, reflected in interpersonal and intellectual processes, such as hallucinations

6. Deficiencies in decision making and ability to make personal choices

7. Self-image changes required by health status

8. Dysfunctional perceptual orientations to health

9. Strains related to life processes, such as birth, growth and development, and death

10. Problematic affiliative relationships.

The nature of phenomena to which the actions of nurses are directed is ascertained by assessment in its various forms, such as observation, interviewing, measurement, and the like. Instruments for the measurement of conditions within the purview of nursing are being developed and tested through nursing research.[16]

Diagnosis is a beginning effort to objectify a perceived difficulty or need by naming it, as a basis for understanding and taking action to resolve the concern. A nurse's conceptualization or diagnosis of a presenting condition is a way of ascribing meaning to it, which may or may not accurately reflect the phenomenon under consideration for treatment. Both the diagnosis and its theoretical interpretation are open to revision; indeed, in some modalities, such as psychotherapy, diagnostic revision is simultaneous with the ongoing therapeutic work.

Theory: Nurses use theory in the form of concepts, principles, processes, and the like, to sharpen their observations and to understand the phenomena within the domain of nursing practice. Such understanding precedes and serves as a basis for determining nursing actions to be taken.

The theoretical base for nursing is partially self-generated and partially drawn from other fields; the resulting insights are integrated into a foundation for nursing practice. Nursing is primarily an applied science: it uses the results of nursing research (which tend to be specifically related to the human responses of concern to nurses) and it selects theories from many other sciences on the basis of their explanatory value in relation to the phenomena nurses diagnose and treat.

The range of theories nurses use includes intrapersonal, interpersonal, and systems theories. Intrapersonal theories explain within-person phenomena. Interpersonal theories aid understanding of interactions between two or more people. Systems theories provide explanations of complex networks or organizations, the dynamics of their parts and processes in interaction. Use of this range of theories is necessary because the various conditions within the purview of nursing cannot be understood in terms of cause-effect relations only, but also require knowledge of system dynamics, pattern and process interactions.

When responses to actual health problems are being treated, the nature of the difficulty and its causes (when known) require theory application for full understanding of extant problems. When responses to potential health problems or maintenance of health are the focus for the nursing action, theories that aid conceptualization of optimal functioning of individual capacities and processes and of the dynamics of human systems are applied to determine reordering of behavior or life styles congruent with healthy living. Thus, theory selected for application in nursing practice is chosen for its relevance to the task at hand.

The ideas and theories of the individual practitioner influence nursing practice in focus and action. Ideally, the actions of the nurse are taken from a theoretical base that includes an accurate understanding of the phenomena in question and a means for evaluation or readjustment.

Actions: The aims of nursing actions are to ameliorate, improve, or correct conditions to which those practices are directed, to prevent illness, and to promote health. Ideally, actions are taken on the basis of understood fact (phenomena). In carrying out nursing care, highly developed technical and interpersonal skills are equally as important as the sensitive observation and intellectual competencies required for the nurse in the nursing situation to arrive at a diagnosis (explanation of a problem at hand) and determination of beneficial nursing actions to be taken. Treatment of a diagnosed condition involves nursing actions that can be described and explained theoretically as to their relation to phenomena and expected outcome

Effects: Nursing actions are intended to produce beneficial effects in relation to identified responses. It is the results of the evaluation of outcomes of nursing actions that suggest whether or not those actions have been effective in improving or resolving the conditions to which they were directed. The results of research study of the relation of particular actions to specific phenomena, determined under controlled conditions, provide more rigorous scientific evidence of beneficial effects to nursing actions than does periodic evaluation or testimonials as to effectiveness.

Nursing values an approach to practice in which investigation and action are interrelated. This approach is apparent in the four characteristics of nursing, which have been described, and is reflected in the use of the nursing process, which serves as an organizing framework for practice.

> The nursing process encompasses all significant steps taken in the care of the patients, with attention to their rationale, their sequence, and relative importance in helping the patient reach specified and attainable health goals. The nursing process requires a systematic approach to the assessment of the patient's situation, which includes reconciliation of patient/family and nurse perceptions of the situation; a plan for nursing actions, which includes

patient/family participation in goal setting; joint implementation of the plan; and evaluation which includes patient/family participation. The steps in the process are not necessarily taken in strict sequence beginning with assessment and ending with evaluation. The steps may be taken concurrently and should be taken recurrently, as in the evaluation of the assessment or the plan of action.[17]

Recognition of the nursing process is reflected in the ANA Standards of Nursing Practice, which apply to all nursing practice. These standards, published by the professional society in 1973, provide one broad basis for evaluation of practice and reflect recognition of the rights of the person receiving nursing care. The standards describe a "therapeutic alliance" of the nurse and the person for whom she or he provides care through use of the nursing process.[18]

The relationship between the characteristics of nursing, the nursing process, and the standards that reflect it are shown in Figure 1. The characteristics of phenomena and theory application are implicit in the standards involving data collection, diagnosis, and planning; that of action is referenced in the standards involving planning and treatment; and the characteristic of effects is related to the standards involving evaluation and revision.

Scope of Nursing Practice

Nursing is a segment of the health care system. In addition to the care an individual provides for his own health, health care is provided through the services of many professions, including nursing, medicine, pharmacy, social work, and dentistry, among others. The term *health care* is therefore not synonymous with nursing care or medical care, but refers to a composite of planned care provided by interdependent professions whose members collaborate with individuals and groups being served. Health care includes many professional segments, each of which has its own definite characteristics and independent functions.

As is true for any profession, the continuity, growth, and thriving of nursing are contingent upon education, research, and administration. Other statements of the American Nurses' Association describe these components of the nursing profession.[19,20,21]

The scope of nursing practice, the contents of the nursing segment of health care, has four defining characteristics: boundary, intersections, dimensions, and core.

FIGURE 1. Defining Chara
Relationship to the Nursing Process

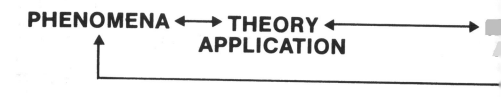

PHENOMENA ⟷ THEORY ⟵
APPLICATION

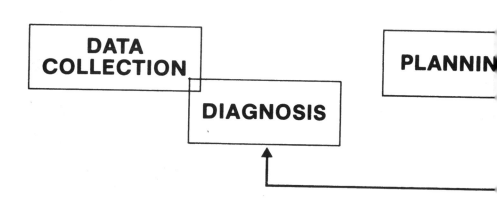

DATA COLLECTION		PLANNIN
	DIAGNOSIS	

I. The collection of data about the health status of the client/patient is systematic and continuous. The data are accessible, communicated, and recorded.

II. Nursing diagnoses are derived from health status data.

III. The plan of nursing care includes goals derived from the nursing diagnoses.

IV. The plan of nursing care includes the priorities and the prescribed nursing approaches or measures to achieve the goals derived from the nursing diagnoses.

V. ▮
pro
clie
par
hea
ma
res

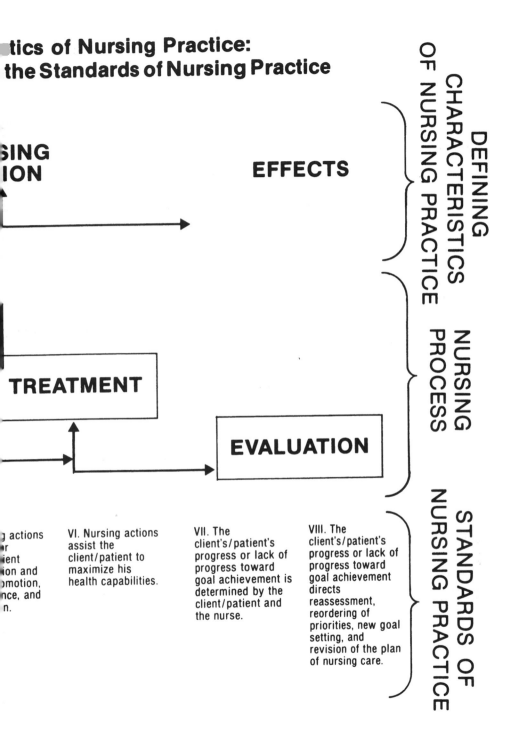

tics of Nursing Practice:
the Standards of Nursing Practice

SING
ION

EFFECTS

DEFINING CHARACTERISTICS OF NURSING PRACTICE

TREATMENT

EVALUATION

NURSING PROCESS

actions
r
ient
ion and
omotion,
nce, and
n.

VI. Nursing actions assist the client/patient to maximize his health capabilities.

VII. The client's/patient's progress or lack of progress toward goal achievement is determined by the client/patient and the nurse.

VIII. The client's/patient's progress or lack of progress toward goal achievement directs reassessment, reordering of priorities, new goal setting, and revision of the plan of nursing care.

STANDARDS OF NURSING PRACTICE

Boundary: The nursing segment of health care has an external boundary that expands outward in response to changing needs, demands, and capacities of society. As is true of all professions, nursing is dynamic rather than static. As new needs and demands impinge upon nursing, and as a consequence of nursing research, the other three defining characteristics of scope begin to change, resulting in expansion of the boundary.

Intersections: The nursing segment of health care intersects with other professions involved in health care. These interprofessional interfacings are meeting points at which nursing extends its practice into the domains of other professions. These intersections are not hard and fast lines separating nursing from another profession; the relations between nursing and medicine at these interfacings are especially fluid and unproblematic in situations in which collegial, collaborative joint practice obtains.[22] All of the health care professions interact, share the same overall mission, have access to the same published scientific knowledge, and in some degree overlap in their activities.

A statement of the scope of nursing ought not to limit the boundary or fix the intersections of nursing with other professions, but should allow for expansion and flexibility. Individual nurses, however, do limit the scope of their practice in light of their education, knowledge, competence, and interest. These differences constitute intraprofessional intersections. All nurses locate themselves somewhere within the scope of nursing on the basis of preparation for the work. Tolerance of differences in interests, in part or whole, and intraprofessional collaboration among nurses serve their shared mission: to promote health.

Core: The core of nursing practice is the basis for nursing care—the phenomena previously described. These conditions are brought into focus by naming or diagnosing them, or by hypothesizing or inferring when the facts are unclear or no diagnosis exists. Diagnosis of phenomena leads to application of theory to explain the condition and to determine actions to be taken—otherwise, diagnosis is mere labeling.

The range of diagnostic categories within the scope of nursing practice is constantly undergoing expansion. The American Nurses' Association, through its five Divisions on Nursing Practice, has identified and is further formulating the phenomena of concern that lie within the scope of responsibility of professional nurses. Various individuals and groups are presently developing classification systems of nursing diagnoses.[23,24,25]

Dimensions: The dimensions of nursing practice are characteristics that fall within and further describe the scope of nursing. A compre-

FIGURE 2. Characteristics of the Scope of Nursing Practice

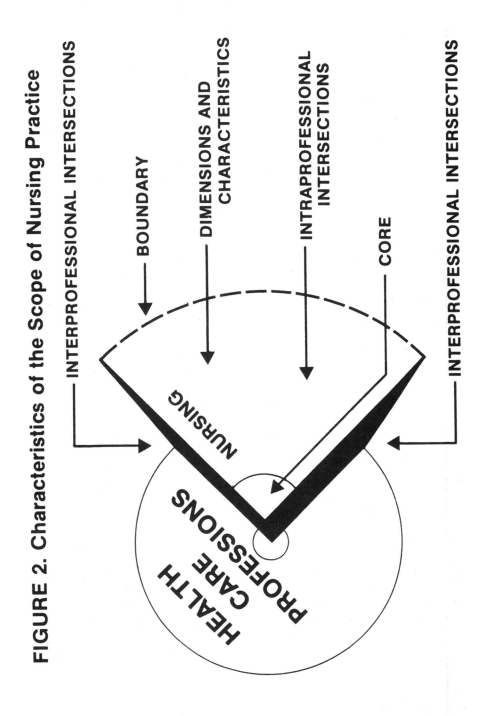

hensive statement of these characteristics would include but not be limited to descriptions of what philosophy and ethics guide nurses; what responsibilities, functions, roles, and skills characterize their work; what scientific theories they use and by what methods they apply them; where and when they practice; and with what legal authority nurses function.

One of the most distinguishing characteristics of nursing is that it involves practices that are nurturant, generative, or protective in nature.[26] They are developed to meet the health needs of individuals as integrated persons rather than as biological systems. The nurturant or nurturing behaviors provide comfort and therapy in the presence of illness or disease and foster personal development. The generative behaviors are oriented to development of new behaviors and modification of environments or systems to promote health-conducive adaptive responses of the individuals to health care crises or problems. The protective behaviors involve surveillance, assessment, and intervention in support of adaptive capabilities and developmental functions of persons. These nurse behaviors are responsive to people with conditions diagnosed and treated by nurses as they apply theory in order to explain and to guide nurse action in practice.

Nurses are guided by a humanistic philosophy having caring coupled with understanding and purpose as its central feature. Nurses have the highest regard for self-determination, independence, and choice in decision making in matters of health. Recognizing that illness and physical handicap tend to erode these attributes of persons, nursing throughout its history has provided health teaching, sharing its expertise with the public through, for example, courses in home health nursing. Presently, nursing is directing its attention to evolving theory and practices focusing on the responsibility of the individual for his own health.

Nurses are committed to respecting human beings because of a profound regard for humanity. This principle applies to themselves, to people receiving care, and to other people who share in the provision of care, as well as to humanity in general.This basic commitment is unaltered by the social, educational, economic, cultural, racial, religious, or other specific attributes of the human beings receiving care, including the nature and duration of disease and illness.

Nursing care is provided in an interpersonal relationship process of nurse-with-a-patient, nurse-with-a-family, nurse-with-a-group. It involves privileged intimacy—physical and interpersonal. Nursing is a laying-on-of-hands practice in which nurses have access to the body of another person in carrying out assessments, comfort care, and definitive treatments. At best, nurses carry out such physical ministrations with compassion and with recognition of the client's dignity. Nursing is a practice in which interpersonal closeness of a professional kind develops and aids the investigation and discussion of problems, as nurse and patient (or family or group) seek jointly to resolve those concerns. Nursing therefore includes an array of functions, including physical care, anticipatory guidance, health teaching, counseling, and the like.

Nursing practice demands professional intention and commitment carried out in accordance with the American Nurses' Association Standards of Nursing Practice and its ethical code. While all nurses are responsible for practicing in accordance with the ANA Standards of Nursing Practice, the level and sophistication of application vary with the education and skills of the individual nurse. Nursing is practiced by nurses who are generalists and by nurses who are specialists. Each nurse remains accountable for the quality of her or his practice within the full scope of nursing practice.

Generalists in nursing provide most of the care for most of the people served by nursing. In other words, in numbers and in amount of service provided, generalists provide the bulk of nursing care. The care provided by these nurses should be available to people wherever they may be at a given point in time and whatever may be their situation in terms of health, disease, illness, or injury at the time. The nurse generalist has a comprehensive approach to health care and can meet diversified health concerns of individuals, families, and communities.

Specialists in nursing are experts in providing care focused on specific clusters of phenomena drawn from the range of general practice. Specialization involves adding to the generic base of nursing practice an organized and systematized body of knowledge and competencies within a discrete area of nursing, applied through specialized practice. Specialized nursing practice represents a refining of interests, either by focusing upon a part of the whole of nursing practice or by focusing upon relations among parts. The phenomena of concerns selected by specialists in nursing practice may relate either to a specialized field or to the interrelation among specialized fields.

All nurses practicing with patients and with persons seeking health address the phenomena that form the core of nursing practice. Variations within nursing practice resulting from differences in level of education, extent of experience, and competence occur in regard to the following:

- Assessment and data collection

- Analysis of data

- Application of theory

- Breadth and depth of knowledge base, especially clinical, psychosocial, and patho/physiological theories relating to nursing diagnosis and treatment

- The range of nursing techniques

- Need for, kind, and extent of supervision by other nurses in practice

- Evaluation of effects of practice

- Identification of relationships among phenomena, nursing actions, and effects (outcomes for the patients).

All nurses are responsible for the inclusion of preventive nursing as part of general and specialized practice. Prevention in nursing is directed to promotion of health and disease prevention; securing prompt attention for medical diagnosis and treatment of disease, or as necessary when predisposition to a given disease is apparent from the nursing diagnosis; and early recognition and management of complications and other consequences due to disease or therapy.

Nurses provide care to people in various states of their life span, from birth through death. Service is provided in environments such as homes, schools, and places of employment, as well as in general and specialty hospitals, ambulatory care settings, skilled nursing facilities, long-term care institutions, protective or custodial institutions, and in newer types of health care settings that are evolving.

All nurses are ethically and legally accountable for actions taken in the course of nursing practice as well as for actions delegated by the nurse to others assisting in the delivery of nursing care. Such accountability may be accomplished through the regulatory mechanism of licensure, through criminal and civil laws, through the code of ethics of the profession, and through peer evaluation.

III. Specialization in Nursing Practice

Specialization is a mark of the advancement of the nursing profession. It suggests that nursing has moved from a global to a more specific way of looking at the field and its practices. Instead of homogeneity (a nurse is a nurse is a nurse), there is a heterogeneity of clinical interests and levels of competence within nursing. Such differentiation, which is a criterion of development, is occurring due to the greater complexity within the whole of nursing practice at this juncture in nursing's history.

Specialization means a narrowed focus on a part of the whole field of nursing. It entails application of a broad range of theories to selected phenomena within the domain of nursing, in order to secure depth of understanding as a basis for advances in nursing practice. It requires identification and more concentrated effort toward resolution of heretofore poorly understood questions related to the phenomena of concern to nurses. It involves empirical and controlled research to clarify aspects of a delimited part of the field of nursing, and to generate refinement of existing nursing practices, or to evolve new ones more likely to be more beneficial to clients or patients.

Specialization arises in five main ways:

- The amount and complexity of knowledge and technology create a demand for a few professionals to give special attention to applications in delimited practice areas.

- A few professional pioneers seek to obtain greater depth of understanding of phenomena related to a segment of nursing and to test new practices intended to correct or ameliorate recognized conditions.

- Public attention and available funds become focused on an area of practice in which heretofore there has been a lack of interest, knowledge, and skilled practitioners.

- The complexity of services exceeds the prevailing knowledge and skills of general practitioners, and this problem is approached by intense personal studies or post-basic study by a few interested professionals.

- Part of a professional field expands, and simultaneously some of its members seek ways for expanded use of their intellectual and other capacities.

Specialization in nursing has been discussed since the turn of the century.[27] Initially, the term *specialist* designated nurses who had graduated from specialized hospitals, or private-duty nurses who worked only with particular kinds of patients. As early as 1910, in ANA convention proceedings, nurses were referred to as specialists. These designations, however, were based upon practical experience or indicated completion of hospital-based "post-graduate" courses in the area of nursing. These courses, which used nurses to provide nursing care but offered little by way of education as it is now known, became so numerous by the early 1940s that the National League for Nursing Education established a committee to study this matter. The committee produced guidelines for advanced courses in nursing.[28]

During the same period, advanced clinical courses began to be offered by various colleges and universities, with the assistance of government funds. The number of nurses holding baccalaureates was exceedingly small at the time, and the university-based advanced courses led to either a bachelor's or a master's degree.

In the 1950s, the meaning of the term *advanced clinical nurse* began to change as universities offered programs for preparation as "clinical specialists in nursing."[29] It was not until the 1960s, however, that all post-basic education for specialization in clinical nursing was provided in graduate programs. By 1980, over 75 colleges and universities offered such programs.[30]

Specialization in nursing is now clearly established. The process has brought about reexamination and revitalization of the generic foundation in which the specialization is rooted. Requirement of the baccalaureate for entry into professional practice, of advanced learning for specialty practice, administration, and teaching, and of doctoral education that includes focus on research capabilities emerges as necessary to fulfillment of nursing's social responsibility.

Specialization in nursing practice assists in clarifying, revising, and strengthening existing practice. It also permits new applications of knowledge and refined nursing practices to flow from the specialist to the generalist in nursing practice and graduate to basic nursing education, thus ensuring progress in the general practice of nursing.

It provides career options, including private practice, for nurses who have particular interests in a part of the nursing field and who seek greater development and use of their abilities as well as increased responsibility and authority in practice. Specialization expedites production of new knowledge and its application in practice. Specialization also provides preparation for teaching and research related to a defined area of nursing.

Criteria for Specialists in Nursing Practice

The specialist in nursing practice is a nurse who, through study and supervised practice at the graduate level (master's or doctorate), has become expert in a defined area of knowledge and practice in a selected clinical area of nursing. Specialists in nursing practice are also generalists, in that they hold a baccalaureate in nursing, and therefore are able to provide the full range of nursing care. In addition, upon completion of a graduate degree in a university graduate program with an emphasis on clinical specialization, the specialist in nursing practice should meet the criteria for specialty certification through nursing's professional society.

Graduate study for preparation as a specialist in nursing practice includes in-depth study of theories relevant to the particular area of specialization and faculty-supervised clinical practice. Faculty supervision means substantial review of data obtained by the graduate student during clinical practice with clients, families, groups, or communities, whichever is required by the focus of the nurse's intended specialization. Such supervisory review is provided on a regularly scheduled basis, over a period of time of sufficient length to provide an in-depth picture of the student's developing competence as a clinical specialist.

Those competencies include ability to observe, conceptualize, diagnose, and analyze complex clinical or non-clinical problems related to health, ability to consider a wide range of theory relevant to understanding those problems, and ability to select and justify application of theory deemed to be most useful in understanding the problems and in determining the range of possible treatment options. Ability to foresee and discuss short- and long-range possible consequences is also to be demonstrated. While this is not an exhaustive list, the foregoing intellectual competencies are of the utmost importance in specialization.

The faculty member who supervises nurses who are preparing for clinical specialization functions as a role model, demonstrating intense interest in the problems germane to the specialty area and expertise regarding the knowledge and practice of that area. Faculty supervisors are also "gatekeepers," permitting only those nurses who achieve a higher level of competence for specialty practice to obtain the graduate degree and recommendation for certification as a specialist. All universities that offer graduate programs in nursing practice should be knowledgeable about requirements for certification of specialists and should inform prospective students whether or not the graduate study to be undertaken is congruent with such requirements.

Certification of specialists in nursing practice is a judgment made by the profession, upon review of an array of evidence examined by a selected panel of nurses who are themselves specialists and who represent the area of specialization.

Specialists in nursing practice thus must meet two primary criteria*: (1) an earned graduate degree (master's degree or doctorate) that represents study of scientific knowledge and supervised advanced clinical practice related to a particular area within the scope of nursing; (2) eligibility requirements for certification through the professional society or completion of the certification process.

The purpose of the criteria for specialists in nursing practice is protection of the public. Unlike generalist nurses, who upon licensure and entry into practice are expected to be competent at least at a *minimum safe level,* specialists are expected to have *expert competence.* The public relies upon boards of nursing, through which nursing practice acts are administered under the authority of state governments, to assure its safety in regard to the general practice of all nurses. Because specialists in nursing practice hold licenses in the state in which they practice, they are subject to the legal constraints and external (outside the profession) regulations that apply under the nursing practice act.

Additionally, however, the public needs clear evidence that a nurse who claims to be a specialist does indeed have expertise of a particular kind. The profession of nursing has a social obligation to the public to satisfy that need, which it does by means of certification of specialists and by accreditation of the graduate programs that educate specialists in nursing practice. These two methods by which the public is protected against false claims are in accord with the prerogative of self-regulation (within the profession) that society has accorded as a trust to its professions. It is in the absence of such within-profession credentialing that the public turns to the law for its protection. Through credentialing of those nurses who claim competence at an expert level, the nursing profession assures the public that these claims of a higher standard of nursing competence are not false.

---

*If these two criteria are insufficient for certain purposes, such as for employment or reimbursement, and especially in the case of a nurse who holds a master's degree but is not certified, still other criteria can be pursued, such as are suggested in the following questions:

1. Was the graduate program *accredited?*
2. In broad outline, what was the theoretical and clinical content of the program, as described in the university *catalogue?*
3. What were the qualifications of the *faculty,* in particular those who taught and supervised the clinical work and therefore were role models? Did these faculty members hold the same or a higher degree than that toward which their students were studying, and were the faculty certified specialists in nursing practice?

Expert competence is an abstraction—the difference between a generalist and a specialist cannot be seen until it has been made concrete through practice, over time; reliance upon credentialing of specialists by the profession is therefore a safeguard for the consumer who uses the services of a specialist in nursing practice.

Role and Functions of Specialists in Nursing Practice

Specialists in nursing practice have autonomy and freedom in practice greater than do nurses in general practice. The autonomy and freedom are based upon broader authority rooted in expert knowledge in selected areas of nursing. This expert knowledge is associated with greater self-discipline and responsibility for direct care practice and for advancement of the nursing profession. The self-discipline includes seeking periodic review of clinical data from an equally prepared expert in the same specialized area of practice.

Nursing is primarily an applied science in that it selects and applies theories from all existing sciences in order to understand and treat those conditions within the scope of nursing. In the last several decades the explosion of knowledge in all scientific fields and the development of nursing research have made monumental the task of theory selection and application in general nursing, and have correspondingly increased the risk of superficiality in this process. Under these circumstances, clinical specialization in nursing has made it possible for some nurses, through graduate-level education, to sharpen their acumen in a designated part of the whole field of nursing.

The effectiveness of the profession is increased when specialists are available to focus their efforts around a particular aspect of clinical nursing, to test application of newly available theory to conditions germane to that clinical aspect, to translate those theory applications into nursing approaches considered more useful than prevailing ones, and to assist in encouraging and speeding up the flow of new knowledge into basic nursing education and generalized nursing practice.

Characteristic functions of specialists in nursing practice include the following:

- Identification of populations or communities at risk

- Direct care of selected patients or clients in any setting, including private practice

- Intraprofessional consultation with nurse specialists in different clinical areas and with nurses in general practice

- Interprofessional consultation and collaboration in planning total patient care for individual and groups of patients, and in planning and evaluating health programs for population groups at risk related to the specialty or the public in general

- Contribution to the advancement of the profession as a whole and to the specialty field.

It is expected of specialists that they engage in a variety of activities consistent with the aims of the specialty and the profession. These activities include the following:

- Selective participation in basic, graduate, and continuing education programs

- Participation in or the conduct of research related to the area of specialization

- Preparation of publications derived from clinical practice and related education or research that would contribute to the general advancement of practice and the profession

- Obtaining certification in the area of clinical specialization through the professional society. Such certification, including periodic review, is the profession's method of assuring the public of the validity of the specialist's credentials.

Legislation to govern specialty practice in nursing should not be sought; all nurses are governed by and liable for practice at the minimum safe levels defined in nursing practice acts. Guidelines for and regulation of practice beyond the basic level of general practice covered by current licensure should be developed within the professional association.

Specialty practice is at the growing edge of the profession, and therefore its nature and scope change as new knowledge develops. Those specialists in nursing practice who continue independent study of the problems within an area, especially through empirical research, experience many changes in role and function.

When nurse specialists are employed in health care settings, descriptions of their position and functions ought not to be standardized. The work rules for the specialist must be jointly determined and negotiated by the applicant and the employing institution. The emphasis should be on developing negotiated positions and organizational arrangements that are most likely to result in freedom and responsibility for maximum use of the abilities of the particular specialist in the particular health care setting. In joint practices and partnerships, in which nurse specialists practice on a private basis with other nurses or other professionals; joint determination of working arrangements and shared responsibility also apply.

Need for Specialists in Nursing Practice

The need of society and the nursing profession for adequate numbers and kinds of specialists in nursing practice should be monitored periodically by the professional society. While the demands of the marketplace should be allowed to regulate excess in numbers, the profession must take steps to assure that universities prepare enough specialists in nursing practice to meet needs for qualified nurse faculty, nurse researchers, and consultants, as well as specialists for direct care practice.

At the same time, the need for specialists must be balanced against the needs of the society and the profession for nurses in general practice. The responsibility of the profession and its specialists for continued strengthening of the generic foundation of nursing is a major one if fragmentation and unjustifiable costs of care are to be avoided in nursing.

Areas of Specialization

The principle applies: *Professional organizations do not initiate trends; rather, they formulate and consolidate those trends already under way within the practices of the professions in society.* Those trends that have been judged to be promising for the advancement of the profession are pertinent to determination of areas of specialization in nursing. Two major social institutions—universities and the American Nurses' Association—are involved in the establishment of areas of specialization in nursing.

Graduate programs that prepare specialists in nursing practice are initiated, established, and conducted by universities, which have the primary social responsibility for the education of scientists and professionals. Among the criteria universities use to decide that an area of specialization in nursing merits establishment of a program are the following:

1. A previously unrecognized area that lies within or would be a reasonable expansion of nursing's scope of practice is identified by one or more nurses or by another person.

2. The nursing faculty at the university has identified through careful study that a sufficient need exists in society or in the health care system to warrant preparing nurses for that new area of specialization in nursing. Nurses who are experts in that area by reason of clinical experience, and who either have or could readily obtain the necessary credentials for academic teaching, are available. Furthermore, the expertise of nurse faculty in the area most closely related to the proposed new one could be co-opted to assist in the design and conduct of the proposed new program.

3. There is ample evidence to believe that the whole field of nursing would be diminished or limited in its long-range aim if the recognized need were ignored.

4. Funds in support of the program are available or could be obtained.

After universities have been providing graduate programs for specialty practice in nursing and accreditation of those programs is in effect, certification of specialists who graduate from those programs becomes a concern of the profession in exercising its responsibility to the public.

The American Nurses' Association has five Divisions on Nursing Practice: community health nursing, gerontological nursing, maternal and child health nursing, medical-surgical nursing, and psychiatric and mental health nursing. These divisions are interest groups; membership in them is open to any ANA member having an interest in a particular division. Each of the divisions offers certification programs for nurses in their respective fields of practice. Thirteen certification programs in nursing practice are currently offered.

Only three of these certification programs are for specialists, i.e. require a master's or higher degree in the area of specialization: the program for clinical specialists in medical-surgical nursing and the two programs for clinical specialists in psychiatric and mental health nursing. Many of the nurses who have been certified in other programs do hold master's degrees in their area of specialization, however, and would be eligible for certification as specialists if such programs existed. Many certified family nurse practitioners, for example, hold master's degrees in their area of specialization that would qualify them as specialists, although the family nurse practitioner certification program does not include a graduate degree among its eligibility requirements.

The ANA divisions on nursing practice also provide councils as opportunities for groups of nurses to meet together and share their interests and concerns related to defined areas of nursing practice.

The American Nurses' Association has recognized that most nursing practice is general nursing in a specialized area, having a specialized population or focus. Within the wide variety of health care institutions, most nursing practice occurs as a concentration in an area of nursing, based on interest, experience, and selection of employment, for example. Additionally, public interest and concern about specific areas of health problems stimulates employment opportunities that sometimes coincide with interests of enterprising nurses. Public concern also sometimes stimulates funds for short-term education of nurses, and the movement toward widespread continuing education for nurses has provided short-term concentrated education. Both of these efforts have been aimed at meeting immediate needs for nurses to work more productively in particular areas of nursing practice. Many nurses with less than graduate education have enlarged their competence for work in such areas without being specialists and without having the recognizable credentials of specialists.

As the professional society for nursing, ANA must provide structural arrangements that recognize the wide diversity of clinical expertise that exists among nurses—generalists, generalists who concentrate their practice in specialized areas, and qualified specialists in nursing practice—and thereby give recognition of and show tolerance for the difference and complexity that characterize contemporary nursing. This diversity must be seen as a constructive response of nurses to social needs in a time of rapid, complex, and sophisticated changes in present-day health care systems.

At the same time, it is incumbent upon the American Nurses' Association to provide for certification of specialists in nursing practice as a means of assuring the public that those nurses who claim to be specialists in nursing practice are so entitled by virtue of holding an earned graduate degree in the area of specialization and meeting the requirements for certification through the professional society.

Within the decades ahead, as a taxonomy of those conditions that nurses diagnose and treat is further refined, new rubrics for emerging clusters of specialization will be formulated within the profession. The American Nurses' Association must be prepared to provide structural arrangements and programming, including certification, congruent with those areas of specialization.

Conclusion

In this statement, nursing and its scope have been defined and issues related to specialization have been presented within the social context in which nurses practice. This social policy statement is intended to assist nurses in conceptualizing their practice; to provide direction to educators, administrators, and researchers within nursing; and to inform other health professionals, legislators, funding bodies, and the public about nursing's contribution to health care.

The statement has defined nursing in terms of the phenomena to which it addresses action (diagnosis and treatment of human responses to actual and potential health problems), its use of theory to guide action, and its evaluation of the effects of action.

It has described nursing's scope of practice in terms of a boundary expanding in response to changing social needs and demands; intersections with the practice of other health professionals; a core that distinguishes nursing from other health professions by virtue of its phenomena of concern; and dimensions that characterize nursing in terms of its practitioners, its practice settings, and its accountability.

The statement has traced the growth of specialization within nursing practice, and has identified specialists in terms of criteria related to graduate education and certification through the professional society.

Nursing's social responsibility has been addressed throughout the statement—in its definition of nursing, its delineation of the scope of nursing practice, and its description of specialization in nursing. The statement is thus both an accounting of nursing's professional stewardship and an expression of its continuing commitment to those its practice serves.

References

1. Page, B.B. Who Owns the Professions? *Hastings Center Report* 5:5 (October 1975), 7-8.

2. Mechanic, D. *Future Issues in Health Care: Social Policy and the Rationing of Health Services.* New York: Free Press, 1979, 6-7.

3. American Nurses' Association Division on Maternal and Child Health Nursing Practice. *A Statement on the Scope of Maternal and Child Health Nursing Practice.* Kansas City, Mo.: the Association, 1980, 5.

4. Antonovsky, A. *Health, Stress, and Coping.* San Francisco: Jossey-Bass, 1979, 123.

5. American Nurses' Association Division on Psychiatric and Mental Health Nursing Practice. *Statement on Psychiatric and Mental Health Nursing Practice.* Kansas City, Mo.: the Association, 1976, 4.

6. Phaneuf, M. *The Nursing Audit: Self-Regulation in Nursing Practice.* 2nd edition. New York: Appleton-Century-Crofts, 1976, 8.

7. Donabedian, A. Foreword, in M. Phaneuf, *The Nursing Audit: Self-Regulation in Nursing Practice.* 2nd edition. New York: Appleton-Century-Crofts, 1976.

8. American Nurses' Association. *Code for Nurses With Interpretive Statements.* Kansas City, Mo.: the Association, 1976.

9. American Nurses' Association Congress for Nursing Practice. *Standards of Nursing Practice.* Kansas City, Mo.: the Association, 1973.

10. American Nurses' Association. *Educational Preparation for Nurse Practitioners and Assistants to Nurses: A Position Paper.* New York: the Association, 1965.

11. Nightingale, Florence. *Notes on Nursing: What It Is and What It Is Not.* London: Harrison and Sons, 1859, preface and 75. (Facsimile edition, J.B. Lippincott Company, 1946.)

12. Henderson, Virginia. *Basic Principles of Nursing Care.* London: International Council of Nurses, 1961, 42.

13. New York State Nurses Association. Report of the Special Committee to Study the Nurse Practice Act, September 24, 1970, 1.

14. New York Education Law (McKinney), Article 139, Section 6902.

15. Kelly, Lucie Young. Nursing Practice Acts, *American Journal of Nursing* 7:74 (July 1974), 1315.

16. U.S. Health Resources Administration. *Instruments for Measuring Nursing Practice and Other Health Care Variables.* 2 Vols. (DHEW Publ. No. HRA 78-53) Washington, D.C.: U.S. Government Printing Office, 1979.

17. American Nurses' Association Congress for Nursing Practice. *A Plan for Implementation of the Standards of Nursing Practice.* Kansas City, Mo.: the Association, 1975, 4-5.

18. *Standards of Nursing Practice, supra.*

19. American Nurses' Association Commission on Nursing Education. *Standards for Nursing Education.* Kansas City, Mo.: the Association, 1975.

20. American Nurses' Association Commission on Nursing Research. *Research in Nursing: Toward a Science of Health Care.* Kansas City, Mo.: the Association, 1976.

21. American Nurses' Association Commission on Nursing Services. *Standards for Nursing Services.* Kansas City, Mo.: the Association, 1973.

22. The National Joint Practice Commission. *Statement on the Definition of Joint or Collaborative Practice in Hospitals.* Chicago: the Commission, 1977.

23. Gebbie, Kristine M., and Mary Ann Lavin (eds.). *Classification of Nursing Diagnoses,* Proceedings of First National Conference. St. Louis, Mo.: C.V. Mosby, 1975, 171.

24. Gebbie, Kristine M. (ed.). *Classification of Nursing Diagnoses,* Summary of the Second National Conference. St. Louis, Mo.: Clearinghouse, National Group for Classification of Nursing Diagnosis, 1976, 200.

25. Gordon, Marjory. Implementation of Nursing Diagnoses (guest editorial), *The Nursing Clinics of North America* 14:3.

26. Bevis, Em Olivia. *Curriculum Building in Nursing: A Process.* St. Louis, Mo.: C. V. Mosby, 1978, 141.

27. Dewitt, K. Specialties in Nursing, *American Journal of Nursing* 1:1 (October 1900), 14-17.

28. NLNE Special Committee on Post-Graduate Clinical Nursing Courses. *Courses in Clinical Nursing for Graduate Nurses: Basic Assumptions and Guiding Principles, Basic Courses, Advanced Courses,* Pamphlet 2. Livingston, New York: Livingston Press, 1945.

29. Burd, Shirley F. The Clinical Specialization Trend in Psychiatric Nursing. Unpublished Ed.D. thesis, Graduate School of Education, Rutgers, The State University of New Jersey, 1966.

30. National League for Nursing Division of Baccalaureate and Higher Degree Programs. *Master's Education in Nursing: Route to Opportunities in Contemporary Nursing, 1979-80.* New York: the League, 1979.

APPENDIX C
TEXT OF THE 1995 REVISION:
NURSING'S SOCIAL POLICY STATEMENT

Reproduced in this appendix are the pages of *Nursing's Social Policy Statement*, the 1995 revision of ANA's 1980 initiating publication: *Nursing: A Social Policy Statement*. That earlier version is reproduced in Appendix B, which starts on page 23.

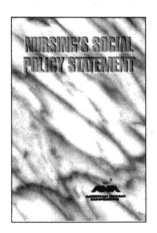

CONTENTS

PREFACE

ursing's Social Policy
Statement, *a reality after several years work by*
hundreds of nurses, represents nursing's
commitment to the society and
people we serve.

Nine nurses served on the task
force that led a profession-
wide effort to create this statement. We are indebted to the
task force members, the
authors of the landmark 1980
Nursing: A Social Policy State-
ment, and to the nurses in
ANA organizational units,
state nurses associations
(SNAs), and nursing organizations throughout the country

who passionately debated the contents and suggested changes after reviewing two drafts of the document.

The task force has responded to widespread suggestions that the statement be both clear and brief. Two areas of compromise contributed to brevity but not always to precision. First, the recipients of nursing care are individuals, groups, families, or communities. This point is made frequently throughout the statement but not in every possible paragraph. We ask readers to keep in mind that nursing practice in its entirety always includes these various recipients of care.

Second, the *individual* recipient of nursing care can be referred to as patient, client, or person. Instead of using all terms or varying terms throughout the document, we chose to refer to individual recipients of care as patients.

The term patient, therefore, is used throughout the statement to provide consistency and brevity, bearing in mind that the terms client or individual, in some instances, might be better choices.

We acknowledge the fact that the term client is preferred by some nurses because it implies a more egalitarian relationship than the term patient. The term client, however, implies that a choice can be made by the recipient of care about which professional, among many, will provide the desired services. At this point in our history, the bulk of nursing practice does not include that type of choice on the part of the recipient of care. The term patient, therefore, is used throughout the statement to provide consistency and brevity, bearing in mind that the terms client or individual, in some instances, might be better choices.

The members of the 1992–1994 and 1994–1996 Congresses of Nursing Practice contributed significantly to the development of *Nursing's Social Policy Statement*. Some helped create the direction and processes for the work, some served on the task force, and all brought insight, commitment, and thoughtful creativity to the consensus-building process. We are grateful for the invaluable support that Dr. Patricia Rowell, Senior Policy Fellow, ANA Department of Practice, Economics, and Policy, provided during public debate on the statement.

Nursing's Social Policy Statement now belongs to the profession. Future congresses of nursing practice will monitor the use of this 1995 statement, aware that the profession, health care, and society are constantly evolving.

Mary K. Walker,
Ph.D., R.N., F.A.A.N.
Chair, Congress of Nursing Practice
1994–1996

Linda R. Cronenwett,
Ph.D., R.N., F.A.A.N.
Chair, Congress of Nursing Practice
1990–1994

INTRODUCTION

ursing's Social Policy
Statement *is a document that nurses can use*
as a framework for understanding nursing's
relationship with society and nursing's
obligation to those who
receive nursing care.

The statement includes
descriptions of nursing and its
knowledge base, the scope of
nursing practice, and the
methods by which the profession is regulated. The conceptualization of the clinical
practice of nursing that is the
focus of this statement will
provide direction for clinicians,

educators, administrators, and scientists within the profession of nursing and inform other health care professionals, public policy makers, and funding entities about nursing's contribution to health care.

This statement is derived from the landmark document, *Nursing: A Social Policy Statement* (1980),[1] the profession's first description of its social responsibility and nursing's roles in the American health care system. The current document presents clinical nursing practice as it has evolved according to society's health needs and sets direction for the future.

The Social Context of Nursing

Nursing, like other professions, is an essential part of the society from which it has grown and within which it continues to evolve. Nursing is dynamic, rather than static, and reflects the changing nature of societal need. Nursing can be said to be "owned by society" in the sense that "a profession acquires recognition, relevance, and even meaning in terms of its relationship to that society, its culture and institutions, and its other members."[2]

This social contract between the broader society and its professions has been expressed as follows:

"Professions acquire recognition and relevance primarily in terms of needs, conditions, and traditions of particular societies and their members . . . societies (and often vested interests within them) . . . determine, in accord with their different technological and economic levels of development and their socioeconomic, political, and cultural conditions and values, what professional skills and knowledge they most need and desire. . . .

"Logically, then, the professions open to individuals in any particular society are the property not of the individual but of society. What individuals acquire through training is professional knowledge and skill, not a profession or even part ownership of one."[2]

The authority for the practice of nursing is based on a social contract that acknowledges professional rights and responsibilities as well as mechanisms for public accountability.

"Society grants the professions authority over functions vital to itself and permits them considerable autonomy in the conduct of their affairs. In return, the professions are expected to act responsibly, always mindful of the public trust. Self-regulation to assure quality in performance is at the heart of this relationship. It is the authentic hallmark of a mature profession."[3]

People seek the services of nurses to obtain information and treatment in matters of health and illness. They use nursing care to resolve problems or manage health-promoting behaviors. Nurses help people identify both short- and long-term health goals and act as advocates for people dealing with barriers encountered in obtaining health care.[4]

Values and Assumptions

Some values and assumptions that undergird *Nursing's Social Policy Statement* are:

+ Humans manifest an essential unity of mind/body/spirit.

+ Human experience is contextually and culturally defined.

◆ Health and illness are human experiences.

◆ The presence of illness does not preclude health nor does optimal health preclude illness.

Furthermore, the relationship between a nurse and patient involves full and active participation of the patient and the nurse in the plan of care and occurs within the context of the values and beliefs of the patient and the nurse. The same values and assumptions apply when the recipient of nursing is a family or community.

DEFINITION OF NURSING

ursing was defined in
Florence Nightingale's Notes on Nursing: What It Is
and What It Is Not, published in 1859, as having
"charge of the personal health of somebody . . .
and what nursing has to do . . . is to put
the patient in the best condition for
nature to act upon him."[5]

A century later, Virginia Henderson defined the purpose of nursing as "to assist the individual, sick or well, in the performance of those activities contributing to health or its recovery (or to a peaceful death) that he would perform unaided if he had the necessary strength, will, or knowledge. And to do this in such a way as to help him gain independence as rapidly as possible."[6] In the 1980 *Nursing: A Social Policy Statement*, nursing was defined as "the diagnosis and treatment of human responses to actual or potential health problems."[1]

These definitions illustrate the consistent orientation of nurses to the provision of care that promotes well-being in the people served. The nursing profession remains committed to the care and nurturing of both healthy and ill people, individually or in groups and communities.

Since 1980, nursing philosophy and practice have been influenced by a greater elaboration of the science of caring and its integration with the traditional knowledge base for diagnosis and treatment of human responses to health and illness. As such, definitions of nursing more frequently acknowledge four essential features of contemporary nursing practice:

+ attention to the full range of human experiences and responses to health and illness without restriction to a problem-focused orientation;

+ integration of objective data with knowledge gained from an understanding of the patient or group's subjective experience;

+ application of scientific knowledge to the processes of diagnosis and treatment; and,

+ provision of a caring relationship that facilitates health and healing.

KNOWLEDGE BASE FOR NURSING PRACTICE

ursing is a scientific discipline as well as a profession.

The knowledge base for nursing practice is derived from multiple sources, including nursing science, philosophy, and ethics, and physical, economic, biomedical, behavioral, and social sciences. To expand the knowledge base of the discipline, nurses generate and utilize theories and research findings that are relevant to nursing practice and fit with nursing's values about health and illness.

Phenomena of Concern

The phenomena of concern to nurses are human experiences and responses to birth, health, illness, and death. Nurses focus on these phenomena within the context of individuals, families, groups, and communities.

Following are examples of phenomena that are foci of nursing care and research:

✦ care and self-care processes;

✦ physiological and pathophysiological processes—such as rest, sleep, respiration, circulation, reproduction, nutrition, elimination, sexuality, and communication;

✦ physical and emotional comfort, discomfort, and pain;

✦ emotions related to experiences of birth, health, illness, and death;

✦ meanings ascribed to health and illness;

✦ decision- and choice-making abilities;

✦ perceptual orientations such as self-image and control over one's body and environments;

✦ relationships, role performance, and change processes within relationships; and,

✦ social policies and their effects on the health of individuals, families, and communities.

The nurse's theoretical and research-based understandings of these phenomena and the preferences of patients, families, or communities guide the formulation of plans of care.

Diagnosis

Nurses identify the human responses to actual or potential health problems they observe and name their conceptualization of the diagnosis using a variety of classification systems.[7] Diagnoses facilitate communication among health care providers and the recipients of care and provide for initial direction in choice of treatments and subsequent evaluation of the outcomes of care.

Interventions

The actions nurses take on behalf of patients, families, or communities are referred to as nursing interventions or treatments. The aim of nursing actions is to assist patients, families, and communities to improve, correct, or adjust to physical, emotional, psychosocial, spiritual, cultural, and environmental conditions for which they seek help.

Nursing interventions may be either direct or indirect. Direct care interventions are performed through interaction with patients. Indirect care interventions are performed away from the patient but on behalf of a patient or group of patients, and are aimed at management of the care environment and interdisciplinary collaboration.[8] Interventions are recommended based on the nurse's clinical judgment about the phenomena of concern and theoretical, practical, or scientific knowledge about the relationships between potential interventions and desired outcomes.

When nursing care is provided to individuals, it is provided within relationships that involve both physical and emotional intimacy. Nursing assessments, treatments, and comfort care are delivered with compassion and respect for human dignity. The interpersonal closeness that develops between a nurse and patient provides a context for open discussion of the patient's experiences of health and illness. The nature of the relationship, therefore, allows the nurse to assist people effectively, whether giving physical care, providing emotional support, engaging in health teaching or counseling, or assisting recovery or a peaceful death.

Outcomes

Nursing interventions are intended to produce beneficial effects for the patient, family, or community. Nurses evaluate the effectiveness of their interventions in relation to identified outcomes and use these assessments to revise diagnoses, outcomes, and plans of care. Whenever possible, recipients of care participate in determining whether nursing actions have been effective.

SCOPE OF NURSING PRACTICE

 ursing involves

practices that are restorative, supportive, and

promotive in nature.[4]

Restorative practices modify the impact of illness or disease. Supportive practices are oriented toward modification of relationships or the environment to support health. Promotive practices mobilize healthy patterns of living, foster personal and family development, and support self-defined goals of individuals, families, and communities.

Nursing's scope of practice is dynamic and evolves with changes in the phenomena of concern, in knowledge about various interventions' effects on patient or group outcomes, or in the political environment, legal conditions, and cultural and demographic patterns in society. The extent to which individual nurses engage in the total scope of nursing practice is dependent on their educational preparation, experience, roles, and the nature of the patient populations they serve.

The extent to which individual nurses engage in the total scope of nursing practice is dependent on their educational preparation, experience, roles, and the nature of the patient populations they serve.

ANA and specialty nursing organizations often delineate scopes of practice for nurses who have chosen to focus their practices in a particular specialty. Differences among nurses in their scopes of practice can be characterized as intraprofessional intersections across which collegial, collaborative practice occurs.

Nursing is not separated from other professions by rigid boundaries. Nursing's scope of practice has a flexible boundary that is responsive to the changing needs of society and the expanding knowledge base of its theoretical and scientific domains.

The boundaries of each health care profession are constantly changing, and members of various professions cooperate by exchanging knowledge and ideas about how to deliver high quality health care. Collaboration among health care professionals involves recognition of the expertise of others within and outside one's profession and referral to those providers when appropriate. Collaboration also involves some shared functions and a common focus on the same overall mission.

Nursing care is provided by nurses in both basic and advanced practice. Within each type of practice, individual nurses demonstrate competence along a continuum from novice to expert.[9] In addition, within each type of practice, nurses can choose to develop expertise in a particular specialty.

Basic Nursing Practice

Nurses who practice at the basic or entry level of practice have graduated from approved schools of nursing and have qualified by national examination for registered nurse (R.N.) licenses. Since 1965, ANA has consistently affirmed the baccalaureate degree in nursing as the preferred educational requirement for basic nursing practice.

Beyond formal education, nurses in basic practice can choose to focus their experience and continuing education on an area of specialty in nursing, and this specialized knowledge base may be acknowledged through certification. As the basis for granting certification, many credentialing bodies require the baccalaureate degree in nursing in addition to other demonstrations of knowledge in specialty practice. Although practices of individual nurses vary according to level of education, experience, competence, and role, all nurses are accountable for meeting the profession's standards of clinical practice. [10]

Nurses practicing at the basic level provide care for patients and families in environments such as homes, schools, and places of employment, as well as in hospitals, ambulatory care settings, skilled nursing facilities, long-term care institutions, protective or custodial institutions, and nurse-managed and other community-based health centers.

Based on outcomes desired, nurses intervene to promote health, prevent illness, or assist with activities that contribute to recovery from illness or to achieving a peaceful death. They may initiate treatments themselves or carry out interventions initiated by advanced practice registered nurses or other licensed health care providers.

Nurses in basic practice are coordinators of care as well as care givers. They integrate the processes of patient service delivery, patient preparation for various tests or procedures, and the monitoring of patient responses to nursing interventions and the interventions of various health care providers.

Advanced Nursing Practice

Advanced practice registered nurses have acquired the knowledge base and practice experiences to prepare them for specialization, expansion, and advancement in practice. *Specialization* is concentrating or delimiting one's focus to part of the whole field of nursing. *Expansion* refers to the acquisition of new practice knowledge and skills, including knowledge and skills legitimizing role autonomy within areas of practice that overlap traditional boundaries of medical practice. *Advancement* involves both specialization and expansion and is characterized by the integration of theoretical, research-based, and practical knowledge that occurs as a part of graduate education in nursing.

As advanced practice nursing evolved in the roles of clinical nurse specialist, nurse practitioner, nurse midwife, and nurse anesthetist, different components or characteristics of advanced practice nursing were adopted. Most nursing organizations and regulatory bodies now recommend or require all the components of advanced practice nursing—specialization, expansion, and advancement—for nurses assuming advanced practice roles.

The nurse in advanced practice acquires specialized knowledge and skills through study and supervised practice at the master's or doctoral level in nursing. The content of study in the specialty area includes theories and research findings relevant to the core of specialization. The expansion of practice skills is acquired through faculty-supervised practice. Certification is sought following completion of the advanced practice registered nurse's graduate study.

Most nursing organizations and regulatory bodies now recommend or require all the components of advanced practice nursing—specialization, expansion, and advancement—for nurses assuming advanced practice roles.

The term advanced practice is used to refer exclusively to advanced *clinical* practice. Nursing practice requires that some nurses assume other advanced roles in the profession—e.g., educator, administrator, and researcher. These roles are critical to the preparation of nurses for practice, the provision of environments conducive to nursing practice, and the continued development of the knowledge base that nurses use in practice. Although nursing educators, administrators, and researchers are prepared educationally at the master's or doctoral level, they are not considered advanced practice registered nurses unless they possess advanced practice knowledge and skills in addition to their expertise in education, research, or administration.

Professions respond to the needs of society by identifying appropriate areas of specialization. As trends evolve and potential new areas of advanced practice nursing are identified, graduate programs are established by universities, the institutions with primary social responsibility for the education of scientists and professionals. Among the criteria universities use to decide that a new area of practice merits establishment of a program are:

✦ The practice area lies within or would be a reasonable expansion of nursing's scope of practice.

✦ A documented need exists for health care in that area of practice.

✦ There is a body of knowledge upon which the practice can be based.

✦ Faculty are available who are expert in that area by reason of clinical experience and expert knowledge.

✦ There is ample evidence that the field of nursing

would be diminished if the recognized need were ignored.

The scope of advanced nursing practice is distinguished by autonomy to practice at the edges of the expanding boundaries of nursing's scope of practice. One hallmark of advanced practice nursing—whether in the primary care setting, the community, or the hospital—is the preponderance of self-initiated treatment regimens, as opposed to dependent functions (i.e., actions taken in response to treatments initiated by other health care providers). Because of the expanded practice and knowledge base, advanced practice nursing is also characterized by a complexity of clinical decision making and a skill in managing organizations and environments greater than that required for the practice of nursing at the basic level.

The scope of advanced nursing practice is distinguished by autonomy to practice at the edges of the expanding boundaries of nursing's scope of practice.

The advanced practice registered nurse works with individuals, families, groups, and communities to assess health needs; develop diagnoses; plan, implement and manage care; and evaluate outcomes of care. Within their specialty areas, advanced practice registered nurses may also plan and advocate care that promotes health and prevents disease and disability; direct care or manage systems of care for complex patient/family/ community populations; manage acute and chronic illness, childbirth, and the care of patients before, during, and after anesthesia; and prescribe, administer, and evaluate pharmacological treatment regimens.

In addition, advanced practice registered nurses serve as mentors, consultants, and educators of nurses in basic practice. They conduct research to expand the knowledge base of nursing practice, provide leadership for practice changes, and contribute to the advancement of the profession, the health care sector, and society as a whole.

REGULATION OF NURSING PRACTICE

 ursing, like other
professions, is responsible for ensuring that its
members act in the public interest in the
course of providing the unique service
society has entrusted to them.

**Professional
Regulation**

The process by which the
profession does this is called
professional regulation.
Nursing regulates itself by
defining its practice base,
providing for research and
development of that practice
base, establishing a system for
nursing education, establishing
the structures through which
nursing services will be delivered, and providing quality
review mechanisms such as a

code of ethics, standards of practice, structures for peer review, and a system of credentialing.

Professional regulation of nursing practice begins with the profession's definition of nursing and the scope of nursing practice. Professional standards are derived from the scope of nursing practice.

ANA, in collaboration with members of its SNAs and members of other nursing organizations:

+ establishes a code of ethics for the profession.

+ establishes a definition of nursing.

+ delineates the scope of nursing practice.

+ establishes standards of clinical nursing practice.

+ promotes the scientific foundations of nursing practice through theory development and research.

+ specifies the appropriate academic credentials for entry into practice at basic and advanced levels, and

+ accredits selected organizations for peer review.

The credentialing boards that are associated with ANA and specialty nursing organizations develop and implement certification examinations and procedures for nurses who want to have their specialty practice knowledge recognized by the profession. Certification is a judgment of competence made by nurses who are themselves practicing within the area of specialization. One component of the required evidence is successful completion of an examination that tests the knowledge base for the selected area of practice. Other requirements relate to the content of course work and amount of supervised practice.

Legal Regulation

All nurses are legally accountable for actions taken in the course of nursing practice as well as actions delegated by nurses to others assisting in the delivery of nursing care. Such accountability arises from the legal regulatory mechanisms of licensure and criminal and civil statutes.

All nurses are legally accountable for actions taken in the course of nursing practice as well as actions delegated by nurses to others assisting in the delivery of nursing care.

Legal contracts between society and the professions are defined by statutes and associated regulations. State nurse practice acts and related legislative and regulatory initiatives serve as the codification of nursing's obligation to act in the best interests of society. Nurse practice acts grant nurses the authority to practice and grant society the authority to sanction nurses who violate the norms of the profession and act in a manner that threatens public safety.

Society is best served when consistent definitions of the scope of nursing practice are used by states: geographic mobility of nurses is enhanced and residents of every state have access to the full range of services that nurses are able to provide. Statutory definitions of nursing should be compatible with the profession's definition of its practice base but general enough to provide for the dynamic nature of an evolving scope of nursing practice.

As advanced practice nursing has evolved, approaches to legal regulation have been based on varying interpretations of societal need and the political philosophies of state constituencies. For both professional and legal regulatory mechanisms, the goal is consistent definitions and criteria for recognition of advanced practice.

Self-Regulation

Nurses exercise autonomy and freedom within their scope of practice. This autonomy and freedom is based upon nurses' commitment to self-regulation and accountability for practice.

One form of self-regulation is accountability for the knowledge base for practice. Nurses develop and maintain current knowledge and skills through formal and continuing education and, where appropriate, seek certification in their areas of practice as a method of demonstrating this accountability.

Nurses also regulate themselves as individuals through peer review of their practices. Peer review is the mechanism by which nurses are held accountable for practice based on the profession's code of ethics. Peer evaluation fosters the refinement of knowledge, skills, and clinical decision-making processes at all levels and in all areas of clinical practice.

CONCLUSION

ursing's Social Policy
Statement *includes a description of nursing in the United
States—the values and social responsibility of the profession,
nursing's definition and scope of practice, nursing's knowledge
base, and the methods by which nursing is regulated. The
statement is both an accounting of nursing's professional
stewardship and an expression of nursing's continuing
commitment to the society it serves.*

REFERENCES

1. American Nurses Association. 1980. *Nursing: A social policy statement*. Kansas City, MO: the Author.

2. Page, B.B. Who owns the profession? Hastings Center Report 5:5 (October 1975): 7–8.

3. Donabedian, A. 1976. Foreword in M. Phaneuf, ed. *The nursing audit: Self-Regulation in nursing practice*, 2nd ed., p. 8. New York: Appleton-Century-Crofts.

4. Pender, N. 1987. *Health promotion in nursing practice*, 2nd ed., p. 27. Norwalk, CT: Appleton & Lange.

5. Nightingale, F. 1859. *Notes on nursing: What it is and what it is not*. London: Harrison and Sons. (facsimile edition, 1946. Philadelphia: J.B. Lippincott Company).

6. Henderson, V. 1961. *Basic principles of nursing care*, p. 42. London: International Council of Nurses.

7. McCormick, K.A., Lang, N., Zielstorff, R., Milholland, K., Saba, V., Jacox, A. 1994. Toward standard classification schemes for nursing language: Recommendations of the American Nurses Association Steering Committee on Databases to Support Clinical Nursing Practice. *Journal of the American Medical Informatics Association* 1:421–427.

8. McCloskey, J.C., and Bulecheck, G. M., eds. 1996 (in press). *Nursing interventions classification (NIC)*, 2nd ed. St. Louis: Mosby Year Book.

9. Benner, P. 1984. From novice to expert: Excellence and power in clir.ical nursing practice. Reading, MA: Addison-Wesley.

10. American Nurses Association. 1991. *Standards of clinical nursing practice*. Washington, DC: American Nurses Publishing.

APPENDIX D
OTHER DEFINITIONS OF NURSING

The historical content of the previous appendices is complemented by these definitions of nursing from other nursing organizations. This international context should help in understanding the new definition of professional nursing in the United States (see page 5) in a manner that better reflects practice in today's complex and evolving healthcare environment.

International Council of Nursing

Nursing encompasses autonomous and collaborative care of individuals of all ages, families, groups and communities, sick or well and in all settings. Nursing includes the promotion of health, prevention of illness, and the care of ill, disabled and dying people. Advocacy, promotion of a safe environment, research, participation in shaping health policy and in patient and health systems management, and education are also key nursing roles.

Reproduced courtesy of the International Council of Nursing.
©2003 International Council of Nursing. Available at http://www.icn.ch/.

Royal College of Nurses (Great Britain)

Nursing is...

The use of clinical judgment in the provision of care to enable people to improve, maintain, or recover health, to cope with health problems, and to achieve the best possible quality of life, whatever their disease or disability, until death.

(See the RCN web site for a PDF file of their publication, *Defining Nursing*, for details and discussion on this definition and its six defining characteristics. http://www.rcn.org.uk/.)

Reproduced courtesy of the Royal College of Nurses.
©2003 Royal College of Nurses.

INDEX

Note – Entries marked by [1980] and [1995] are from the 1980 and 1995 versions of ANA's nursing social policy statements. The page numbers of these entries are from this edition, not the original publications, which are both reproduced in Appendix B (1980) and Appendix C (1995).

A

Advanced Practice Registered
  Nurse, 8, 10
    [1995] 77–79
    expanded skills, 9
      [1995] 77
    specialized skills, 9
      [1995] 77–79
Advanced roles in nursing, 10
    [1995] 77–79
    See also Specialization
American Nurses Association
  (ANA), *vi*, 2, 8, 9, 12
    [1980] 27, 39, 42, 54, 55
    [1995] 75, 76, 81
    Congress on Nursing Practice
      and Economics, *vi*
      [1980] 26
    fundamental documents, 19–21
Assumptions of nursing's social
  contract, 3
    [1995] 66–67

B

Basic nursing practice, [1995] 76–77
Bill of Rights for Registered Nurses,
  2, 21

C

Certification, 9, 11, 12
    [1980] 34
    [1995] 76, 81
    See also Licensing

Certified Nurse Midwife, 9
Certifed Nurse Practitioner, 9
Certified Registered Nurse
  Anesthetist, 9
Clinical Nurse Specialist, 9
Client (term), *v*, 22
Code of ethics for nurses, *vi*, 11, 12
    [1980] 34, 45, 46
    [1995] 81
    timeline of development, 19–21
Collaboration with other healthcare
  professionals, 8
    [1980] 32–33
Consumer (term), *v*, 22
Contract between nursing and
  society, 1, 2, 3, 6, 13
    [1980] 33–34
    [1995] 65–66
Coordination of care, 8
Credentialing, 9, 11, 12
    [1980] 34
    [1995] 76, 81
    See also Licensing

D

Decision-making, 7, 11
Definitions of nursing, 5, 6, 12, 13
    international, 87
    [1980] 35
    [1995] 68–69, 81
Diagnosis
    [1980] 37, 42
    [1995] 72

E

Education, 8, 10, 11, 12
  [1980] 34
  [1995] 78–79
Emotional care, 7
Environment, 7
Error reporting, 11
  See also Regulation
Essential features of nursing, 5
  [1995] 69
Ethics, *vi*, 11, 12
  [1980] 34, 45, 46
  [1995] 81
  timeline of code, 19–21
Evidence-based practice, 7
Expanded skills, 9
  [1995] 77

H

Health promotion and teaching, 7
Healthcare policy, 3, 11
Healthcare system, 3, 6, 7
Henderson, Virginia, 5

I

Interventions, 7, 8
  [1995] 72–73, 76

K

Knowledge base, 7–10, 11
  [1995] 70–73

L

Legal issues. *See* Regulation
Licensing, 9, 13
  [1980] 46
  See also Certification

N

Nightingale, Florence, 5
Nurse administrator, 10
Nurse educator, 10
Nurse policy analyst, 10
Nurse researcher, 10
Nursing
  advanced roles, 10
  basic practice, [1995] 76–77
  collaboration with other
    healthcare professionals, 8
    [1980] 32–33
  contract with society, 1, 2, 6, 13
  [1980] 33–34
  [1995] 65–66
  definitions of, 5, 6, 12,
  13, 87, 88
  [1980] 35
  [1995] 68–69, 81
  definition. *See* definitions
    of nursing.
  education, 8
    [1980] 34
    [1995] 78–79
  essential features, 5
    [1980] 40–41
    [1995] 69
  key issues, 7
    [1980] 29–32
    [1995] 71
  knowledge base, 7, 8, 11
    [1995] 70–73
  place in society, 1, 8
  research, 7, 12
    [1980] 34
    [1995] 70
  scope of practice, 8–9, 12
    [1980] 35–46
    [1995] 74–79

Spiritual care, 7
Standards of nursing practice, 8, 12
    [1980] 34, 39, 45
    [1995] 81
    timeline of development, 19–21
State nursing practice acts, 13
    [1980] 34, 35
    See also Regulation
Supportive practices, [1995] 74

T
Terms for recipients of nursing care,
  v, 22
Theory. *See under* Nursing

V
Values of nursing's social
  contract, 3, 7
    [1995] 66–67